Caring for mentally ill people

Caring for mentally ill people

Psychological and social barriers in historical context

ALEXANDER H. LEIGHTON
Dalhousie University

CAMBRIDGE UNIVERSITY PRESS

Cambridge
London   New York   New Rochelle
Melbourne   Sydney

Published by the Press Syndicate of the University of Cambridge
The Pitt Building, Trumpington Street, Cambridge CB2 1RP
32 East 57th Street, New York, NY 10022, USA
296 Beaconsfield Parade, Middle Park, Melbourne 3206, Australia

© Cambridge University Press 1982

First published 1982

Printed in the United States of America

Library of Congress Cataloging in Publication Data
Leighton, Alexander Hamilton, 1908–
Caring for mentally ill people.
Includes bibliographical references.
1. Mental health policy – Nova Scotia –
History – Case studies. 2. Community mental
health services – Nova Scotia – History – Case
studies. 3. Mental health policy – Case studies.
4. Community mental health services – Case
studies. I. Title.
RA790.5.L38   362.2′1′09716   81–38486
ISBN 0 521 23415 8 hard covers   AACR2
ISBN 0 521 28816 9 paperback

To Jane M. Murphy

Contents

Acknowledgments

The case study of a psychiatric service that underlies much of this book was the work of a number of individuals who collaborated in data gathering and analysis. Victor G. Cardoza assisted in founding the service and sat on its Advisory Board and, subsequently, on its board of directors. Through twenty-one years he was an astute observer, and he has been a major source of both data and interpretive ideas during the analysis.

Alice L. Nangeroni participated administratively during the early years of the service, developed a system for collecting and recording its activities that has formed a major component in the case study, and conducted a systematic survey (aided by W. D. Longaker) of public attitudes toward the service. James L. Tyhurst initiated the idea of a case study at the time the service was founded. Cardoza and Nangeroni have each reviewed the manuscript several times and made numerous suggestions for improvement.

Benjamin K. Doane has been a sharp critic, has encouraged expanding the work beyond the original case study design, and, as head of the Department of Psychiatry at Dalhousie University, has been a generous provider of many facilities and a source of much encouragement.

Preliminary organization and qualitative analysis of the case study materials was conducted by Jean Himmelhock and Sharon Schwartz under the direction of Sandra Rasmussen. Herbert L. Levine visited all the mental health centers in Nova Scotia with a view to collecting materials that would give perspective to the case study. E. R. Rosenberg aided in planning the analysis.

An extensive search and review of the literature pertaining to the history of mental hygiene and mental health movements was conducted by Ralph Kuna, who suggested also a number of highly valuable interpretations. Linda Pereira and Debbie Murphy assisted in examining various other aspects of current literature.

Consultants who reviewed the manuscript or responded to queries on particular points included Wm. O. Aydelotte, Robert Belliveau, Douglas

Black, John Black, Donald Brennan, Ray Carlson, Felix Doucet, Bogdan Erjavec, Jerome Frank, Wm. Gore, Jack Griffin, R. O. Jones, Khaliq-Kareemi, Gerald Klerman, Douglas Lewis, Philippe LeBlanc, Clyde Marshall, Milton Mazer, John McCleave, Peter New, Hector Pothier, Alexander Richman, Milton Sabshin, Richard Snyder, Zebulon Tainter, Ralph Townsend, and Leon Trakman.

Indefatigable work in preparing the manuscript for publication was done by Vivian Crowell, Jocelyn Fraser, and Joanna Greene. To all of these I wish to express my deeply felt personal appreciation and most sincere thanks.

Grateful acknowledgment is also made to Health and Welfare Canada for grants 602-7-148(29) and 603-1042-22(48). These supported the qualitative and quantitative analyses, the review of the literature, and the preparation of the manuscript. The founding of the service and the Stirling County Study research related to it were supported by a number of sources. Special mention is made of Cornell University, the Department of National Health and Welfare Canada, the Nova Scotia Department of Public Health, the Carnegie Corporation of New York, the Milbank Memorial Fund, the Ford Foundation, and the National Institute of Mental Health of the U.S. Public Health Service – grants MH08180 and MH12892.

The Russell Sage Foundation made a notable contribution by supporting the Nangeroni survey of local reactions to the service at the end of its first five years.

Alexander H. Leighton

1   Introduction

The project to be reported in the following pages is one in which a research effort profoundly modified the body of theory that gave rise to it. The research consisted of a case study about the first twenty-one years of a small, rural mental health service, The Bristol Mental Health Centre in Stirling County, Nova Scotia (throughout this book, code names have been used for most towns and counties in Nova Scotia and for the Centre, itself), together with epidemiological investigations of the population it served. The body of theory dealt with mental illnesses and the structure and functioning of society. It was centered on questions of how social, cultural, and psychological factors might affect the origin, course, and outcome of mental illnesses and the services aimed at the treatment and prevention of mental illnesses. On the basis of this body of theory, my colleagues and I founded the Centre in 1951, planning to show that the great majority of people with mental illnesses could best be treated in their own communities, that preventing mental illnesses and promoting mental health were feasible goals, and that the involvement of community members in such a program would not only strengthen the program but would also increase the ability of the community to recognize and cope more effectively with many of its psychological and social problems.

The results of the research suggest not so much that the theories were wrong (although some were) as that they were insufficient and did not take into account many factors of major importance. For instance, the number of persons in the population with complaints and disabilities of the kinds commonly treated by psychiatrists and clinical psychologists was far greater than was first supposed; also, the local management of community affairs was far more compromised, because of transcommunity networks of often competing powers and special interests. The concepts of *mental illness* and *community* both turned out to be deficient because of imprecision and lack of generally agreed-upon meanings. Thus, our body of theory proved to be in many ways an unsatisfactory guide to program development and led to disappointments in goal

1

achievement. At the same time, however, the case study shed light on what was wrong with the theories and pointed to areas where growth, refinement, and additional information were needed.

If one goes back to the origins of modern psychiatry at the close of the eighteenth century and traces what happened subsequently, it is apparent that there has been a succession of movements concerned with the care, control, and prevention of mental illness. These movements have included moral treatment, mental hospital development, mental hygiene, psychoanalysis, child guidance, and, in our own time, community mental health. Each has combined very high levels of expectation with very modest levels of achievement. Thus, across almost two centuries, a wave pattern is evident: hope and activity, followed by disillusionment and turning away. It is as if each movement had had its rise blocked by a low, invisible ceiling against which it vainly struggled until exhausted.

In view of this history, it would seem that the story of the Bristol Mental Health Centre is but one among many such stories and that it exemplifies themes that are very old and very widespread. Two books published in 1978 lend credence to this idea: the *Report to the President*[1] from the President's Commission on Mental Health, and *Today's Priorities in Mental Health*[2] from the Vancouver Congress of the World Federation for Mental Health. Both call for reaching more mentally distressed people, treating them with more compassion, adjusting treatment to individual needs, eradicating stigma, creating opportunities for personnel to develop themselves, providing community supports, emphasizing prevention, coordinating services, and extending scientific knowledge.

These were among the main goals that concerned us in 1951, and they were also goals that had been advocated long before – some as far back as the eighteenth century. Their vigorous reiteration in these recent, comprehensive, stock-taking books requires an explanation. Why, after so many years, do we still hear urgings similar to those of Philippe Pinel, Dorothea Dix, and Adolf Meyer?

It is important to realize, of course, that, despite recessions of action and interest, some progress has been made. Treatments for mental illnesses are now much more successful than formerly. Equally important, services today are within the reach of a much larger proportion of people. There is also widespread recognition that mental illnesses are common and that stigma is something that ought to be overcome. Compared to the state of affairs at the end of the eighteenth century, all these facts stand out. Much of the advance, furthermore, has come about during the last fifty years.

On the whole, however, the cumulative impact of all the various movements is more noteworthy for its small size than for anything else. The major efforts to cope with mental illnesses seem largely discontinuous; they illustrate Dahrendorf's dictum that "history proceeds by changing the subject" rather than through developmental stages.[3]

The purpose of the present book is to describe some of the main social and psychological factors that interfered with achieving the goals of the Bristol Mental Health Centre and that were not sufficiently taken into account in our original body of theory. Much of what will follow has been difficult for my colleagues and me to accept because it has required us to modify, and in some instances reject, ideas in which we had considerable confidence. It is possible that a part of what I shall say will appear to the reader as unduly harsh criticism of well-meaning people in the mental health movement – people who were doing the best they could under difficult circumstances. I do not wish, however, to attack good intentions, for I believe them to be in too short supply almost everywhere today. Nor do I intend to be hard on individuals. My aim, rather, is to look at ideas that have not worked, at ideas that have not been sufficiently tried, and at the underlying responsible social and psychological processes. Inasmuch as I have in the past shared much of the thinking characteristic of the mental health movement, the book can be seen largely as self-criticism.

The core of the book is derived from the case study of the Bristol Mental Health Centre, together with some descriptive epidemiological data, presented in the broader context of a historical review and interpretive analysis. To give the full case study is unfeasible because of the amount of material and undesirable because an emphasis on individuals might obscure the main purposes of the book. We must recognize, of course, that there is a price to be paid for avoiding direct reference to individuals. For example, some of my points will not be supported by the best illustrations available or, on occasion, by all the facts that might have been adduced to back them up. To some extent I have tried to compensate by drawing support for certain points from the literature rather than from the case study.

The social and psychological factors that will concern me in the course of the book are divisible into two categories: those intrinsic to the mental illness field and those extrinsic to it. By "mental illness field" I mean the phenomena of mental illnesses, all ideas about them, and the principal actors involved with them, such as patients, their relatives, clinicians, nurses, social workers, administrators, and others. The intrinsic factors, therefore, are those that are inherent in theories about the nature of mental illnesses, in programs for treatment, in attitudes toward people who are mentally ill, and so on.

The extrinsic factors, which often have a major impact on the intrinsic factors, are those that are inherent in the larger society in which the mental illness field is imbedded. These include episodic phenomena such as wars, economic depressions, immigrations, rapid cultural change, and sociocultural disintegration. Others are the more steady, chronic patterns of malfunction that prevail in human organizations generally and that affect not only medical and public health services but also educational and welfare systems, all branches of government from federal to local, private industries, and voluntary associations. As far as the Western world is concerned, history makes it plain that, from the Greek city states to the present, human societies have rarely achieved a high level of skill in self-management and have never succeeded in making it stable. Mental hospitals, community clinics, federal bureaus, schools, private companies, prisons, and town governments have many defects in common – for instance, lack of clear, generally understood goals and lack of a dependable system of rewards for doing a good job. In the course of this book, I shall first try to describe the intrinsic factors, in order to provide a foundation, and then move on to some of the extrinsic factors.

The data employed in the case study consist of clinical records, policy and planning memoranda, annual reports, files of correspondence, minutes of staff meetings, minutes of Board of Directors meetings, and financial records of the Bristol Centre. Because a formal case study was planned from the beginning, this material is extensive and detailed.

Personal observations noted at various times and recollections also form a part of the data. These come mainly from Judge Victor G. Cardoza and myself. We were participants in the policies and operations of the Centre from its inception and have collaborated in much of the analysis.

The conceptual orientation of the book is psychiatric in a medical and clinical sense, although I hope not narrowly so. It is based on the frame of reference presented in *My Name Is Legion*.[4] Anthropology and sociology have exerted considerable influence, not only because of their general relevance, but also because I have conducted research in these fields and have tried to apply some of their orientations to the tasks of bringing about or ameliorating social changes.[5] I have, accordingly, been concerned with theories of structure and function, social deviance, labeling, cultural relativity, and culture and personality.

In striving to integrate explanatory ideas and empirical observation, I have found short-range theories more useful than highly developed systems, be they psychoanalytic, anthropological, or sociological. My emphasis is, thus, on descriptions of phenomena and on interpretations that are closely related to the observable.

The audience I should like to reach consists of policymakers, planners, and program developers who are directly concerned with mental illnesses and mental health. Included are those who make political decisions and their advisors, the boards of mental health centers and hospitals, professionals in mental health services, and the members of voluntary associations that focus on the improvement of mental health. It is my hope, however, that there may be still others who will find the book of interest, such as teachers and students in psychiatry, public health, and the behavioral sciences as applied to health.

2   Barriers to effective mental health care

In order to come to a set of central points as quickly as possible, I shall begin by describing some conclusions and reserve most of my presentation of evidence for later chapters. These conclusions pertain to the intrinsic social and psychological factors mentioned in the previous chapter that hinder the development and maintenance of both treatment and care. They comprise exceedingly numerous vectors, which are tightly interactive in the complex manner of all life processes. It is, however, possible to organize the tangle in one's mind as a scheme composed of four great barriers to treatment and care, each with numerous subsidiaries. This representation, like other efforts to confine nature to a scheme, is in many ways a caricature, but it can, perhaps, serve to make a mazy topic more graspable and to highlight aspects that are deserving of attack.

Barrier one: the heterogeneity of "mental illness"

"Mental illness" is not something that is scientifically defined but is rather a residual category into which medical and societal events have, in the course of history, precipitated a great variety of human disorders that have little in common except misery for the patient, behavior that troubles other people and persistence. Consider, for example, that the categories range from brain syndrome through psychoneurosis to personality disorder; that the causes include many different combinations of genetic, traumatic, infectious, nutritional, degenerative, psychological, societal, and cultural factors; that syndromes vary widely in the degree to which the causes are dependably known, with general paresis at one extreme and personality disorders at the other; that the degree of disability ranges from slight to total; that dangerousness ranges from none to great; that duration runs from transient situational disorders to life-long psychoses; that frequency in populations ranges from the rare *fou savant* to exceedingly common patterns of anxiety and depression; and that treatability

6

extends from good responses to reassurance and medication to intracta-
bility in the face of every known remedy.

Such multidimensional, nonlogical heterogeneity is fatiguing for the
mind to grasp. One is tempted to drop distinctions, lump together disparate matters, generalize, and oversimplify. This makes thinking and communication seem easier, but it misrepresents reality, creates errors in
judgment, and distorts the transmission of information. In consequence,
conceptualization, planning, provision of services, practice, the conduct
of research, and public discussion about the state of the field all suffer.

Such troubles are augmented by the employment of pseudo-unitive
terms as, for instance, *mental illness* (when used in the singular) and *mental health*. These are confounding terms with enormous power to mislead
because of their many different, and sometimes contradictory, meanings
and especially because of their synecdoche. The movement toward deinstitutionalization, for example, has been obfuscated and at times rendered
malignant by people thinking in terms of "*the* mentally ill" rather than
differentially about kinds of mental illnesses, degrees of disability, and
varying needs for varying types of care. The results have often been cruel-
ly inappropriate, much as a vast, headlong campaign to digitalize *the*
heart patient would be.[1]

It can be argued that when people speak of mental illness they really
know very well that the referent is heterogeneous and are only employing
the words for convenience in a summary sense. This is doubtless often so,
but it commonly happens that speakers and hearers lose sight of the quali-
fication. In using lump words, they slip into lump thinking about mental
illnesses and make policies, plans, and programs as if they were dealing
with a single illness that had a coherence more or less like tuberculosis.[2]

Such lump thinking is encouraged by the practices whereby those interested in mental health mobilize public support. Like other special-interest groups, they employ slogans for rallying purposes that are almost
always expressive of lump thinking. Indeed, the more lump a slogan, the
more universal its appeal and the more support it is likely to gain. The
disadvantages appear later, when goals have to be defined and steps
toward their accomplishment specified. The participants then find agreement and consistency difficult because they lack the necessary mutual
understanding, and often have incompatible goals.

Barrier two: the emotions stirred by mental illness

Although, in and of itself, the heterogeneity of mental illnesses makes
thought and communication difficult, the difficulty is increased several

magnitudes by the capacity of some mental illnesses to arouse emotions that can develop great intensity and assume protean forms. The intensity reaches peaks from time to time without regard to facts, reason, or balanced judgment; and the forms range from revulsion to compassion.

Emotions of this sort were evident in the atrocities committed against mentally ill persons in the name of demon and witchcraft beliefs during the Middle Ages. We like to think that with the Enlightenment of the eighteenth century there came a swing away from superstitious cruelty to scientific humanitarianism. Yet emotions continued to surge in recurrent waves, sometimes as blind enthusiasm, sometimes as blind indifference, and sometimes as blind hostility. Thus, our humanitarian scientific era has actually included not only moral treatment and child guidance but also the use of large hospital oubliettes and gas chambers and the indiscriminate discharge of seriously ill persons to shift for themselves in populations that are little prepared psychologically, organizationally, or economically for their reception. Multiform, changeable, and contagious emotion has made it extremely difficult, even for professionals, to agree on and adopt a coherent and rational approach by which to deal with the heterogeneity described as barrier one.

One could argue that all diseases seen as chronic and life threatening or incurable make people uneasy, and I would accept this general uneasiness as a component in the emotions inspired by madness. There probably is some common ground with the feelings once aroused by leprosy, syphilis, and tuberculosis and still aroused by cancer. But I think that the response to insanity has additional dimensions of intensity and irrationality. There is something particular in these disorders that evokes in human beings existential apprehension that is akin to the fear of the dead and of ghosts, demons, trolls, and other apparitions. That something, I believe, is incomprehensible behavior. Madmen and madwomen are perceived as unpredictable and therefore as uncanny and dire.

I think, further, that much indirect evidence in support of a theory of inherent dread of insanity can be adduced from sources such as research on animal behavior (attack on the oddly behaving one), studies of social evolution, and cross-cultural comparisons. The plausibility of the theory was borne in on me in the course of my observations during our case study of the Bristol Mental Health Centre. To pursue this topic, however, would be too great a digression. I shall content myself, therefore, by expressing the view that if one considers the stigma of mental illness to be nothing more than ignorance, lack of humane feeling, cultural bias, or, "not understanding," then one is underestimating the strength of the enemy.

No doubt some people will feel that the notion of inherent dread is defeatist because it implies that nothing can be done about the stigmatization of mentally ill persons. This is not a necessary conclusion. There are many inherencies that are modifiable. Cats can learn to behave in a friendly way toward mice; humans can learn to fly, to live under water, and to participate in numerous other activities that run counter to innate tendencies. What the theory means is that overcoming stigma is this kind of problem and that it needs to be recognized and tackled as such.

The notion of inherent dread can alert us to the presence of classic defense mechanisms. For example, awareness of the existence of mental illnesses, like awareness of the fact of death, can be *repressed,* and this repression can be aided by burying patients out of sight in isolated institutions; or, mental illnesses can be *denied* and the denial rationalized by theories of "normal" responses to defects in "our society";[3] or, the apprehension can be *sublimated* by such devices as turning mental illness into mental health; or, there can be *displacement,* whereby the anger inspired by the dread comes to bear on those concerned with caring for mentally ill persons.

Uneasiness about mental illnesses can also be mitigated by a sense of intellectual mastery. On such a basis we can explain, at least in part, the grip on the public mind attained by some theoretical notions, and also why they often become stripped down to simplistic forms that have the sole merit of being easily grasped by almost anyone. At this stage, they are generally represented by slogan words or phrases that mobilize strong emotions; "organic," "genetic," "unconscious drive," "social role," and "our culture" are academically toned examples, whereas "scientology" and "primal scream" exemplify others.

Barrier three: insufficient use of science

Barrier one and barrier two in conjunction lead to barrier three. The blend of extreme heterogeneity of subject matter with strong, unstable, multiform emotional reactions has made the steady growth of scientific work exceedingly difficult. Notable investigations have, of course, been carried out, particularly in chemotherapy, neuroregulators, and genetics. Less has been achieved, however, in the study of clinical, social, cultural, and psychological phenomena. In these areas, the theory-building aspect of the scientific process has commonly far outrun the theory-verifying aspect, thus following in the footsteps of Leibnitz rather than Newton.[4]

Barrier three may be considered as having, itself, three major divisions, all closely interrelated. The first is the lack of a frame of reference for the mental illnesses that can guide and unite research, policy, and planning. The second is the difficulty of initiating and maintaining a volume of research sufficient to bring about major advances in understanding. The third is a parallel difficulty, that of utilizing the research once it has been done.

Frame of reference

A frame of reference is a coherent arrangement of knowledge and near knowledge, including observations, theories, assumptions, and guesses, and it is served by a standardized terminology that distinguishes clearly among these components. As one important function, it must keep in the forefront of consideration the differences between what can be considered true and what must be seen as tentative, or not yet known. Most scientific fields have fairly clear frames of reference about which nearly all participants agree (even though they may disagree about theoretical points within the frame) and in terms of which they shape their teaching, their practice, their research, and their policies. Such frames are altered in response to increments of scientific information as these are generated, but they are, at least ideally, impermeable to other influences.

The contrast to this in the mental illness field is obvious. Instead of a frame of reference, we have a fluid mix of innumerable ideas, many incompatible with each other and often charged with overwhelming feeling. They range from belief in the nonexistence of mental illnesses through psychodynamic formulations and therapeutic heuristics to biogenetic models. The technical language reflects this state; imprecise and deficient in standard meanings, it lacks the ability to distinguish between observable phenomena and inferred constructs. This semantic confusion extends even to such basic concepts as *affect*.[5]

Far from having a frame of reference that is resistant to influences other than the scientific, the mental illness field is highly susceptible to fashionable ideas that spring from perturbations in society at large. These are always represented as progress, a moving away from out-of-date notions to improved insights and truer understandings. But it is change itself (marked by such prestigious words as *creative* and *innovative*) that carries weight, not objective evidence. While they are current, furthermore, the fashionable ideas tend to be ideological rather than theoretical, tentative, and disprovable. With metaphysical, metapsychological, and mystical properties, many of them can be easily linked to magical, religious, and salvationist cults.

The absence of a frame of reference means that the mental illness field is not only heterogeneous but also amorphous, with indefinite internal partitions and outer boundaries. Many of its disparate components have conceptual margins that overlap, interpenetrate, and meld with each other. Then, too, efforts at theory building are often all-inclusive – for example, the application of psychoanalytic theory to normal as well as abnormal psychological processes, Meyer's attention to "normal psychobiologic adaptive problems,"[6] and Rennie's definition of social psychiatry as being concerned "not only with the mentally ill but with problems of adjustment of all persons."[7] Those who make such efforts are justified insofar as they say that psychiatry can increase our understanding of man. Their views lead to error, however, when "can increase" is mistaken for "has increased" and especially when it is believed that psychiatry has some special edge in this regard over other disciplines. Such ideas can easily become delusions of omniscience. As Rumke says:

Don't you know that . . . an understanding of neurosis is, in itself, an understanding of man? I retort, But no, that is exactly what I do not accept . . . one who understands neurosis does not necessarily understand other illnesses, nor the man in good health.[8]

One inhibiting consequence of the panhuman orientation in psychiatry has been a downgrading of nosology and a discouragement to objective, phenomena-based classification.

Competition among the various disciplines of the medical, social, and behavioral sciences that have interests in mental illnesses has further augmented the difficulties of achieving a frame of reference. What emerged in the thirties, and especially during World War II, as a promising forward thrust of interdisciplinary cooperation,[9] has since then very largely broken apart in Balkan wars over treatment territories and monopolistic theories.[10]

There has also been a plague of false issues. Questions about the use of words, for example, are mistaken for questions about the nature of things. "Is a whale a fish?" is a question of word usage. The answer depends on what one means by a fish; and without a standard definition of fish it is unanswerable. An old-time whaler and a zoologist could never agree, because fish means something different to each. "Does a whale have lungs and breathe air?" is a question about the nature of things and is answerable through scientific procedures.

Debates over whether homosexuality or mental retardation are mental illnesses constitute word-usage issues, but they are often mistaken for questions about the nature of things and posed as if there were a correct scientific answer. One can well argue on a scientific basis that these two conditions are different from schizophrenia or psychoneurosis and, hence, should have different terms and be regarded differently. To argue that they are or are not mental illness, however, is to flounder in the logically absurd, as long as mental illness has no generally accepted definition.

In a more optimistic vein, let us observe that if one gives up trying to think of mental illness as a unity and turns instead to its major component constellations of behavior patterns, one can see that some of these are beginning to be surrounded by fairly solid frames of reference. Schizophrenia, affective psychosis, and drug and alcohol abuse constitute some examples. Even psychoneurosis and personality disorders are much more conceptually manageable when each category is considered as a possibly independent set of phenomena.

Volume of research

The problems of motivation and resources for conducting an adequate volume of research are old ones, having been with us since the beginning of the modern humanitarian and scientific orientation 200 years ago. The history of Philippe Pinel's ideas is a case in point. Pinel is well known for his advocacy of moral treatment and his reform of hospital care. He is less well known for his insistence that his, or any other, theory should be assessed by scientific procedures. As quoted by Lewis,[11] Pinel states in the second edition of his *Traité* in 1809:

A continual comparison must be made of the proportion that obtains between recoveries and admissions, at different times in the same place or in different hospitals over the same period of time. If the comparison is to be sound, several requirements must have been satisfied: namely, extreme care in supervising the manner in which registers are kept and tables constructed; regular notes compiled with particular detail on those patients who leave the hospital apparently recovered; and precise figures for the number of recoveries, and relapses, and, of course, failures. The elementary mathematics of probability should be applied to the analysis of these data.

The task was too big for one man, and Pinel was unable to inspire the necessary interest in a sufficient number of his followers. It is only today that a beginning is being made toward the implementation of these goals. Even so, we are still far short of what he envisioned.

Moral treatment itself, on the other hand, became popular without benefit of scientific evidence and was transformed into an ideology maintaining that all mental illnesses were curable if caught in time – the "cult of curability." It played a significant part in the great mental hospital movement spearheaded by Dorothea Dix and inspired claims of 90- and even 100-percent cure rates. As we shall see in the next chapter, the movement lost its appeal soon after the middle of the nineteenth century. Notions of biological determinism began to dominate so that, ultimately, the cult of curability was replaced by an incubus of incurability.

The point to note for our purposes is that the decline of belief in moral treatment was as much without scientific support as was its rise. From today's perspective, it seems likely that moral treatment did, indeed, make a considerable difference to some kinds of patients. The need to ascertain just what it could do, however, was overlooked in both the period of enthusiasm and the period of disillusionment.

The nonscientific pattern illustrated by moral treatment has recurred again and again through the years in a great variety of contexts. Most recently, it has been manifest in the community mental health center movement, in efforts to "prevent mental illness," and in programs for deinstitutionalization.

Utilizing research

To illustrate the problem of utilizing the results of scientific research, we may turn to epidemiology. By the 1950s, a number of studies had reported total prevalence rates of mental illnesses in populations that were much higher than was generally supposed. For instance, in his study of Berlevåg, in Norway, Bremer gave a total of 22 percent at least somewhat impaired for all persons over the age of ten.[12] Essen-Moeller's investigation of Lundby in Sweden shows a prevalence rate of 26 percent impaired when his figures are adjusted to the same age range and to diagnostic categories that approximate those of Bremer.[13] Shortly afterward, our study in rural Canada produced a figure of 20 percent in need of psychiatric attention for persons over seventeen years of age,[14] and Srole et al. in New York reported 23 percent impaired among persons between the ages of twenty and fifty-nine.[15]

These and other total-prevalence figures, coming as they did from such disparate sources, implied a need for rethinking psychiatric concepts and also a confrontation for policymakers interested in developing adequate services for mentally ill persons. The treated prevalence rates were rarely much over one percent,[16] meaning that, if the total-prevalence studies were correct, for every individual receiving such a service, there were some twenty more who also needed attention.

So large a discrepancy could not be overcome by increases in personnel and service units without running into overwhelming manpower problems and prohibitive costs. Grappling with the issues raised by the epidemiological studies, therefore, would have involved reconsidering the prevailing definitions of mental illnesses,[17] reassessing goals, redesigning services, reassigning professional roles, creating new patterns of training, recruiting auxiliary aides, and so forth. For policymakers and educators, it was easier to disregard the epidemiological findings than to face such prodigious changes. Their reaction was very much like that of the wife of the Bishop of Worcester when she heard that Mr. Darwin had discovered that men were descended from monkeys: She hoped it was not true, but if it were true she certainly hoped that word of it would not get around.

For many years, the findings were ignored, and the main effort to meet service needs continued to be through multiplying conventional service units. By the mid-sixties, ideas about new designs began to emerge, and the community mental health center movement took shape but there was still insufficient attention to the size and nature of the task as adumbrated in the epidemiological studies. Today, at the beginning of the eighties, the magnitude of the discrepancy has become evident as a result of failures and shortfalls, so that virtually everyone is now aware that changes must come in the way services are delivered and in the distribution of tasks among professionals, paraprofessionals, and others. This realization, however, could have been foreseen and not bought at such a very high price in terms of human suffering and wasted resources.

My point is not that the epidemiological findings should have been accepted at their face value and at once made the basis of new policies. It is rather that they should have stimulated extensive new policy-oriented research aimed at verification and clarification. Then the lessons that have since come from hard experience might have been learned earlier and in a more humane fashion.

Barrier four: extensiveness – too many goals and too few priorities

The cumulative effect of barriers one, two, and three is to create a fourth barrier that might be characterized as "extensiveness." The array of goals, intentions, and activities in the field of mental illness are of such vast proportions that accomplishment is defeated. From the mental hospital movement of the nineteenth century to the mental health center movement of our own time, there have been repeated efforts to achieve goals that were beyond what society could or would sustain.[18] These efforts have had bloom and blight properties, with initial enthusiasm and high expectation being followed by disappointment and loss of public confidence, leading to bewildering reversals of policy and the abandonment of mentally ill persons. Commonly, it was and is the chronically ill individual who endures the brunt of these changes.[19]

The rise-and-fall pattern can be analyzed in terms of three interactive sets of factors: (1) the large number of people with mental illnesses; (2) the small number of people with appropriate training and motivation for giving them care; and (3) the cost of quality care.

As we have just noted, the moral treatment and mental hospital movements suffered from a swing of popular and professional fancy to biological determinism. This, however, was only part of the disaster. The hospitals were overwhelmed by numbers of patients far in excess of their capacity,[20] to which was added a succession of major economic depressions in North America and Europe after 1870.[21]

It is scarcely necessary to point out the parallel that exists today in community mental health centers and other related services. The hopes and ambitions of the mental health movement run counter to demands for cost containment and to the spirit that animated Proposition 13 in California.[22] Both the experience of the past and the exigencies of the present draw attention to the need for clear priorities. Without these, programs tend to fly high and then fold, and it seems extremely probable that, in the end, there is a falling short of what could have been accomplished.

Staff deficiencies and other lacks have, in various configurations through the years, undermined not only state and provincial hospitals but also mental hygiene clinics, child guidance clinics, and community mental health services. The insufficient numbers of capable and motivated people have resulted in compromises and substitutions that have sooner or later worked badly, leading to the neglect, mismanagement, and injury of patients. The existence of mental hospital "snake pits" and "cuckoo's nests" has been a popular theme (sometimes unjustly so), but there has not been comparable recognition that outpatient services also suffer from ignorance, indifference, overenthusiasm, and lack of technical training, and that these can also injure patients. Here, as well as in the hospitals, inappropriate psychological guidance and insufficiently controlled use of medications lead to suicides and to damaged brains, kidneys, and cardiovascular systems.

As Grinker[23] noted some years ago, overreaching in the mental illness field calls to mind Lord Ronald, the Stephen Leacock hero who flung himself on his horse and "rode madly off in all directions." The essence of the Lord Ronald syndrome can be described as coequal strivings for goals that are not coequally feasible and that are, in any event, too numerous for achievement with available resources. The result is that the goals appear pitted against each other in a competitive struggle for limited funds and manpower, thus mutually interfering with one another while dissipating the resources.

Deficiencies in terms of money and personnel for this or that program have, of course, been frequently recognized. But such recognition is usually at a tactical rather than a strategic level, and the common response is to try to raise more money, expand training, and recruit more vigorously. Such actions are usually powered by a faith that force of effort alone will overcome the difficulty. The experience of the last 175 years shows, however, that by and large this is not so.

Those of us who are enthusiasts for the control and prevention of mental illnesses, like other enthusiasts, commonly regard those who oppose us as malign. Yet the core of the issue – the generally overlooked core – is not willingness to give versus mean selfishness, or humane concern versus brutal indifference, real as these are. The core of the issue is the management of limited resources, of making choices among many different kinds of humane goals, as well as among objectives that are necessary for human survival. Overpopulation, poverty, malnutrition, child mortality, displaced people, crime, nuclear control, environmental pollution, and national defense are only a few of the other great problems that absorb money and qualified personnel.

In addition, there is the philosophical, ethical, political, economic, and practical question of how great a burden, and how much interference with self-realization, should be imposed on healthy and competent persons for the benefit of those with psychological handicaps. Whatever the answer, it certainly does not include the word *unlimited*. If effort is not to be squandered, and if credibility is not to be destroyed by failures, the Lord Ronald syndrome must be replaced by a stable system of priorities.

3 A glance at history

The existence of the four barriers discussed in Chapter 2 and their power to obstruct are evident across most of the last 200 years. This chapter endeavors to provide a glimpse of them in historic context. It also tries to show the background from which developed the goals that became a focus of the Bristol Mental Health Centre in 1951.

Moral treatment and the mental hospital movement

Human habitation in North America is believed to go back at least ten thousand years. European landings probably began with the Norsemen, followed a few centuries later by major waves of the Spanish, French, British, and others. It is unlikely that mental illnesses were absent among any of these different kinds of people. The Algonkian languages, no less than the European, contain the concept of insanity and vocabularies for dealing with it. For example, in Micmac *eloowawea, eoonusea,* and *aweiea* all mean insanity.[1] According to one of the earliest Norse accounts of an attempt to establish a settlement south and west of Greenland, the colony dissolved because its leader, Freydis, an illegitimate daughter of Eric the Red, had delusions and committed mass murder.[2] And the pilgrims on the Mayflower were sorely troubled by an insane crew member.[3]

Among settlers and Indians alike, it is probable that the social institution that did most of the caring for mentally ill persons was the family. This pattern was common throughout the world, with supplemental care-taking provided, to some extent, by religious institutions such as monasteries and hospices. Gradually, however, as the culture of the West became more urbanized, and as feudalism receded, town and/or parish authorities began to accept some responsibility for mentally disabled persons who had no effective kin or who were too disturbed for family management. There were parallel changes in ideas about the nature of mental illnesses. Those afflicted ceased, by degrees, to be seen in a context of

17

saints, witches, and demons and were seen more in the context of the unfortunate, the wretched, and the ill.

The rise of humane concern

The nineteenth century witnessed, both in Europe and in North America, the rise of humane concern for mentally ill persons, initiated by thoughtful and sensitive people such as Chiarugi, Pinel, and Tuke, who were affected by the hideous custody under which deranged persons were often forced to live. The spirit of the movement is symbolized by Robert Fleury's well-known painting of Pinel ordering chains removed from patients in a Paris asylum.

This trend was part of a larger one that, building on origins in the Enlightenment of the eighteenth century, gave attention to the conditions of the poor, the orphaned, the handicapped, and the powerless.[4] Writers like Wordsworth, Dickens, and Hugo prompted questioning of the comfortable view that poverty was preordained and challenged the reader's conscience while wringing his heart. Encompassing the romantic period's emphasis on feeling, and suffused with the optimistic belief that the world could and should be made a better place, the movement saw, before it spent itself, numerous social reforms, such as the repeal of the corn laws, the Catholic emancipation, and the abolition of slavery. It was a factor in the 1848 revolutions in Germany and France, in the partnership of Marx and Engels, and in the application of the ideas of Adam Smith.

The period was also one in which public health came into being as an expression of public conscience. Its spirit of putting thought into action is expressed in the life of Rudolf Virchow, one of its founders. Virchow, who was a physician with major discoveries in pathology to his credit, went into the Prussian Parliament in order to fight for the poor – and against Bismarck.[5]

The origins of the mental hospital movement

The ideas of Pinel and Tuke led from the initiation of moral treatment to what may be called the great mental hospital movement. This was animated by the beliefs that mental illnesses were curable, that the environment was all-important, and that mental hospitals could be created so as to provide a therapeutic environment. Such an environment would consist in a staff with humane understanding of each individual patient and a regime that was kind but firm, building healthy minds and healthy bodies; it would contain a balance of work, exercise, and recreation; there would be music, religious services, lectures by distinguished speakers, and a constant encouragement to develop wholesome thinking. Patients would thus become restored to their dignity as human beings, to their self-control, and to their self-confidence.[6]

The world outside the hospital was considered a bad place for the mentally ill, a place that at best prevented recovery and at worst did harm through promoting organic disease and the inculcation of evil habits.[7] It seems probable that hospital treatment was seen as something like the care of a fracture. A broken leg is put in a cast for protection and to allow healing, and the patient is supported by good food, good general medication, and friendly care. It was thought that if the mentally ill person was brought into a hospital early enough and was separated from the evil and damaging influences of society, he or she would be certain to recover and able to return to the dangers of the world with defenses and coping abilities restored.

It is interesting to note that moral treatment was, in some respects, a version of family treatment, or at least modeled on such care as could be given by a wealthy family with a large house, land, extended kin, and numerous retainers. Many of the hospitals and retreats were on estates similar to those maintained by European nobles and distinguished North American families. The superintendent was the kindly, all-powerful father who ate in a dining hall with the estate's inhabitants, welcomed them to his house, presided at musical evenings, and involved his wife and children in a total commitment to creating and demonstrating a physically, psychologically, and socially healthful way of life for the benefit of the patients. It is said of Dr. Samuel Woodward of Worcester Hospital in Massachusetts "that when patients arrived at his institution, manacled and caged, he would greet them and personally free them from their restraints. He would then escort them into the dining room and seat them beside his family at the head table, as a symbol of the patient's expected return to normal social functioning."[8]

The mental hospital movement, like later movements, was strongly charged with emotions that had roots in political, philosophical, and religious imperatives. In the views of some people, salvaging the mentally ill was a demonstration of the mysterious resources of the human mind and soul and of the power for good and evil inherent in the way people treated and guided each other – that is, in social forces. The belief in the curability of mental illness was tied to ideas about the nature of all minds and about the human capacity for growth – spiritual and intellectual.

The results claimed for moral treatment were not, in the beginning, unrealistic. Pinel, for instance, mentioned that one-third of the patients were cured during 1798 and 1799 at Chareton.[9] As the hospital movement grew and took shape, however, the percentage of cures rose to fifty and then to eighty and even a hundred percent.[10] It is evident that the proponents of the movement, being convinced of the rightness of their views, built expectations higher and higher. Large sums of money were thus mobilized, at first from private donors and popular subscriptions and then, later, through the formation of tax-supported hospitals.

Opposition to the mental hospital movement

A current counter to the mental-hospital movement set in shortly after mid-nineteenth century and soon became a tide. Public interest and support waned as disbelief in the curability of mental illnesses grew. Many hospitals became overcrowded, understaffed, and underfinanced, and, in some of them, conditions evolved that were just as bad as those that had aroused the revulsion of Pinel and Tuke more than fifty years before.[11]

Numerous reasons can be adduced for this shift, some of them inherent in the changing nature of Western society itself. It is possible that the Crimean and Franco-Prussian Wars in Europe and the Civil War in the United States did much to undermine optimistic humanism and faith in ideals. Darwin's theory of organic evolution shook the churches and was interpreted by some people to mean that mankind was not and could not be more noble than an ape.[12] The concept that species differentiation was generated by the survival of the fittest raised questions about the social wisdom of preserving the weak, the incompetent, and the insane. And the rise of industry, it has been claimed, led to the spread of materialistic values at the expense of humanitarianism, as the struggle "to succeed" resulted in the apotheosis of self-centeredness at the expense of altruism.

An additional set of ideas that had a direct impact on the care of mentally ill persons came from the contributions of science to medicine through the identification of a number of specific etiological agents such as the anthrax and tubercle bacilli. Reasoning by analogy, theories of biological determinism took on the force of dogma, and with this came a disposition to feel that kindly, custodial care was the best society could do for mental patients while waiting for science to uncover specific causes and specific cures. Notions of social-environmental cause and social-environmental treatment were given scant room in this frame of reference.

As in our time, there were also countertrends to scientific and secular values, doubtless stimulated, as they are now, by increasing uncertainties about traditional religious beliefs. A major one of these trends was spiritualism, which reached a degree of popularity, even among the educated, that is little recalled today. One contemporary observer, Templeton Strong, a lawyer, stated:

What would I have said six years ago to anybody who predicted that before the enlightened nineteenth century was ended hundreds of thousands of people in this country would believe themselves able to communicate daily with the ghosts of their grandfathers? – that ex-judges of the Supreme Court, senators, clergymen, professors of physical sciences, should be lecturing and writing books on the new treasures of all this . . .

It is surely one of the most startling events that have occured for centuries and one of the most significant.[13]

Trends and movements of this sort are not only antiscientific in their values but are also apt, as in some groups today, to regard mental illnesses as a nonproblem. One of the spiritualist leaders likened spirit communications to the recently completed Atlantic cable; there was, he said, at that very moment a great jubilee in the spirit world, similar to the "renaissance" that was then developing on earth. Soon these two great gatherings of mortals and spirits would meet as one in a gigantic reunion of the past and the present until all time would be as one and death would be no more. Clearly, this vision allowed no forms of illness.

Economic troubles also greatly increased for the mental hospitals when, as noted in Chapter 2, a series of severe depressions began in 1871 and lasted until 1900.[14] Custodial care, especially if trimmed down to bare physical essentials, was far less expensive than a therapeutic environment. Biological determinism, therefore, had a strong appeal to political leaders and policymakers anxious to please a tax-paying electorate. It provided them with formidable justification for denying funds to mental institutions.

While this was happening, many hospitals near the East coast of North America were overwhelmed by admissions as a consequence of massive immigrations from Europe. The city populations were rapidly inflated far beyond expected growth rates. The immigrants, furthermore, had a considerably higher rate of admission to mental hospitals than the native born.[15]

Over and above changes in society that adversely affected the mental hospital movement, the movement itself contained flaws that led to its destruction. Chief among these was the belief that hospital treatment inevitably cured mental illnesses. Conviction about this was both profound and sweeping, yet was substantiated by little that could be called scientific. Neither *mental illness* nor *cure* were adequately defined but, on the contrary, meant different things to different people. Although there were, of course, those who were temperate in their claims and who pointed out that some kinds and stages of illnesses were more likely to respond than others, there can be little doubt that curability was oversold by the enthusiasts. One critic, for example, has argued that the denominator enthusiasts used when claiming recovery rates of over 80 percent was the number of patients discharged, not the number of patients admitted.[16]

What actually happened in the course of time was that the proportion of chronic ("incurable") patients gradually increased, occupying more and more of the hospitals' space, like sediment silting the channels of a river. The facilities for providing environmental treatment were thereby reduced and, thus, denied to those patients who could benefit from them and be returned to a more normal way of life. The program for moral treatment was therefore, in part, scuttled by its failure to take into account the reality of chronic illness. Hospital discharge rates dropped,[17] and disillusionment and reaction followed on overexpectation and unrealizable hope.

The problem of the chronically ill was not overlooked by everyone. The Willard Hospital in New York state was opened in 1869 expressly for the care of such persons. Its establishment, however, produced an explosion of emotional protest and a decade of debate. The protest had to do with such issues as costs and administrative feasibility, but it also rested on compelling resistance to the idea that some patients could not be cured.[18]

The enthusiasm for curing mental illnesses through the hospital environment had several other effects that also helped to undermine the mental hospital movement. One of these was disregard of cost. To quote Grob, "At the outset, the major emphasis was placed upon securing the necessary funds to open, the construction of the physical plant, and the problem of making the institution operational as quickly as possible."[19] Expectations of a 100 percent cure rate must have made the problem seem much less formidable than it turned out to be when the discharge rates began to fall far short of this. The movement's need for money increased, which made it exceedingly vulnerable to the economic depressions from 1871 onward.

A parallel difficulty was that the moral-treatment programs required large numbers of highly trained and highly motivated staff members, of whom there were actually very few. The momentum and enthusiasm of the mental hospital movement rolled onward, nevertheless, creating institutions and erecting buildings far ahead of society's personnel resources or its ability to create training programs to supply them. The result was recurrent trouble stemming from staff incompetence and staff turnover.[20]

The combination of overcrowding, underfinancing, and inadequate staffing produced stagnant and brutal institutions with the lawful regularity of the moon, sun, and planets producing the tides.

If the mental hospital movement had risen in a wave of enthusiasm that had very little scientific evidence to support it, its decline was equally uninfluenced by scientific data. The convictions that mental illness was incurable and that mental patients would never recover were also sentiments[21] without factual support. On the basis of our present-day understanding, it seems likely that the moral-treatment procedures were effective with some patients, perhaps very effective with many patients. A great deal might have been learned through a systematic examination of what was actually happening and follow-up studies of the outcomes – in short, through following Pinel's original suggestions as quoted in Chapter 2.

Although the movement undoubtedly brought help to numbers of people suffering from mental illnesses, it also did harm: It made promises it could not keep, taught fallacies about the nature of mental illnesses, and created programs for which it could not obtain sufficient, stable resources in terms of either funds or personnel.

The mental hospital movement in Nova Scotia

Let us turn now from the broad view to a more highly magnified one of a part of this history. The province of Nova Scotia is appropriate for our scrutiny both because it exemplifies many of the general trends of the time and because its particular story is the background for our case study.

The beginning in Nova Scotia was the creation of the Public Hospital and the Orphan House in Halifax in 1750, a year after the founding of the city. As pointed out in Chapter 2, reform or innovation is not usually a simple struggle of the new, good, and energetic against the old, evil, and slothful but is rather a tangle of tensions over how to divide society's finite resources and over who shall have the advantages desired by many. In the present instance, the government originated the idea of financing the orphan house, at least in part, by depriving the troops of their rum allowance and applying the money thus saved to the new institution.[22]

The hospital and orphan house were followed in 1752 by a building to house paupers and criminals. In 1758, a bill was passed to establish a new asylum for the poor. Legislation in 1759 provided that "if any persons be idiots or lunatics or sick or weak they should be taken care of by the keeper" of the asylum. In 1812, a wing was added "for the care of lunatic persons" and thus inaugurated in Nova Scotia the idea of more specialized attention for the mentally ill. All these facilities, however, proved inadequate to the population's needs and the asylum was soon serving as a home for the indigent and aged, a general hospital, a sailors' hospital, an orphans' home, and a lying-in institution, as well as a lunatic asylum. Conditions were apparently frightful, for it was said about 1832 that in "one garret over the ward . . . there were 18 beds, nearly in contact, in which 47 persons were nightly crowded."[23]

The Nova Scotia version of the great mental hospital movement can be seen as beginning in Halifax when a group of citizens, headed by Hugh Bell, a leader in the legislature, sought the creation of a hospital especially for mental patients. In 1844, Bell, while mayor of Halifax, contributed a year's salary as the nucleus for a fund. Dorothea Dix, at that time North America's leader in the mental hospital movement, was drawn into the endeavor and, in 1850, presented a memorial to the provincial legislature in which she stressed the curability of those treated early and the cut in costs that would result. She also selected the site and made contributions to the planning of the hospital. The cornerstone of Mount Hope (now the Nova Scotia Hospital) was laid in June 1856, and, the first patient was admitted toward the end of 1857.[24] The creation of this institution marks the transition in Nova Scotia from a custodial orientation to one of treatment and expectation of cure.

Mount Hope was scarcely completed, however, before the decline began. Reduction in staff occurred before the first twelve months had run their course,[25] and over the next decade the progressive ideas and plans for moral and environmental treatment gradually gave way to the reality of custody. The struggle then became one of trying to make that custody reasonably humane. Lack of motivated, dependable, and appropriately trained personnel caused it to be a very hard struggle. "The difficulty of finding suitable guardians" is mentioned again and again in the hospital's reports.

The swelling of the population by immigrants was not such a problem in Halifax as it was in Boston, New York, and other East-coast cities. Nevertheless, the admission rates were higher than expected. In 1876, the superintendent of the hospital, Dr. James R. DeWolfe, analyzed the census data for Nova Scotia and reported that from 1851 to 1871 the population had increased 40 percent, whereas the number with severe mental illnesses had increased 169 percent. He also noted that, while there were 318 patients in the Nova Scotia Hospital, there were an estimated 1254 in the province.[26]

Tension about costs in the hospital became strong, spurred no doubt by the economic depressions that have been noted as beginning in 1871. That the legislature's Committee on Humane Institutions charged Superintendent DeWolfe with extravagance in the management of feeding and heating[27] may have been an expression of this. By 1884, there were difficulties in getting the municipalities of the province to pay for those of their residents who were patients in the hospital; according to the commissioner of public charities, "A very urging letter was sent to each municipality last year, but as the receipts show, without any appreciable effect."[28]

In the latter part of the century, the problem posed by chronic, "incurable" and indigent patients was approached through the creation of "municipal mental hospitals" throughout the province. These were, in essence, county homes, and the intent was to have local areas assume responsibility for the care of their own mentally ill residents and so reduce the drain on the provincial government. Some parallels to the philosophy of the deinstitutionalization movement of the 1970s are evident.

The municipal hospitals, however, were no sooner established than serious complaints began. With regard to one, for instance, the inspector of humane institutions said in 1892:

No language of condemnation is too strong to use towards the officials responsible for the thoughtless indifference displayed with reference to the water supply in the institution. For years the women [i.e., the patients] have been obliged to climb up a ladder to the top of the tank and down another on the inside of it to the water – when there is any – and return with a full bucket by the same route with the water required for the cooking and washing of fifty people. During the dry spells, when the tank is empty the supply is carried in buckets from a neighbouring farm.[29]

It is instructive to look at the figures representing patient populations at the close of the century and to consider them in light of the expectations of those who had initiated the mental hospital movement in Nova Scotia some sixty years previously. Dix's memorial to the legislature emphasized the view that cases treated early in the course of mental illness were cured and those neglected became incurable. Thus, although the "expense of a patient under Hospital treatment is greater than in Almshouses or at private charge, the ultimate expense is much less than if they are enforced to become incurable, and so remain a life-long burthen." She further added that "the malady of insanity, when brought under *early, efficient* treatment, is, except there be organic disease, equally manageable and curable as a fever or a cold." At the end, she dared the legislature "to *refuse* what you *know* will heal the sick."[30]

In the twelve months ending on September 30, 1900, there were 401 patients in the Nova Scotia Hospital. In the course of the year, 127 had been admitted and 102 discharged. The discharge figure was composed of 26 who died, 6 who were considered unimproved, 19 improved, and 51 cured. Compared to the total admitted, the last figure amounts to a cure rate of 40 percent; cured and improved combined came to 55 percent.[31]

The number of insane persons in the municipal mental hospitals as of September 30, 1900, was stated to be 586, and, given the nature of these institutions, it is reasonable to think that these were virtually all chronic and disabled cases.[32] If we make an arbitrary guess and assume that half of those in the Nova Scotia Hospital were also chronic and disabled, this would mean that out of 1089 cases under institutional care during the twelve months prior to September 30, 1900, 837 were chronic and disabled and only 252 had some possibility of recovery or improvement under the conditions then existing.

These figures are far short of the expectations that drew the mental hospital movement forward. Dix and her colleagues would likely assert that this was because of failure to provide *"early, efficient* treatment." Given the way hospital care evolved, there is justification for such a claim, and it can be argued that a better recovery rate could have been obtained with sufficient financial and staff resources and that, further, the growth of the belief in the incurability of mental illness worked as a self-fulfilling prophecy.

It is not, however, plausible to suppose that these factors explain all the patients who failed to recover. It seems likely that there really were a considerable number of mentally ill persons who could not be "cured" in the hospitals or in any other social or psychological environment, no matter how ideal. Some of the patients, for example, must have been suffering from schizophrenia, which is not "as curable as a fever or a cold." Others undoubtedly had paresis (syphilis of the brain). Modern knowledge of genetics and the evidence from cross-cultural studies in psychiatry indicate the occurrence of some schizophrenic and depressed conditions that, although they may be helped, are rarely "cured" through environmental manipulation. The patient figures, I think, reflect these factors, among others, and illustrate how the channels for care giving became "silted" by long-staying and disabled patients, with a corresponding reduction in treatment resources available to those who had the potential for recovery. The sweeping nature of the mental hospital movement's belief in curability fostered inadequate planning for the chronically ill.[33]

This brief review of the mental hospital movement in Nova Scotia points up a number of well-documented themes pertinent to the hindrances noted in Chapter 2, including the emotional intensity that bypasses or distorts data-based evaluations, the underestimation of chronicity of some mental illnesses, the underestimation of costs and staffing requirements, and the overestimation of the willingness and/or ability of society to care for people with mental illnesses. These factors led to results that did not match the promises of the movement. Instead, they intensified its vulnerability to the economic depressions, the rise of belief in biological determinants, and the increase in the number of persons for whom admission to mental hospitals was demanded.

It would seem that progression from the demonism of the Middle Ages to the reason of the Enlightenment did not remove insanity's capacity to invoke awe, dread, mystery, and the possibility of miracle. Rather, the cult of curability through hospital care can be seen as a belief in miracles in a new form – rationalized, but still akin to exorcism. It is evident that the mystery of insanity continued to invite ontological speculations that had no horizons. It stimulated questions about the meaning of dreams, nightmares, intuition, delusions, inspiration, hallucinations, ecstasy, and melancholy, some or all of which any person could share with mentally ill persons. Doors were thus opened to questions not only about the human mind but about the nature of reality and God – vistas that, in their vastness, are both terrifying and alluring and that lead easily to explanatory legends and intuitive convictions.[34]

Such a combination of emotion and philosophy made it very hard for people in the mental hospital movement to develop agreed-upon definitions and to carry out systematic observations according to standard procedures, in short, to conduct scientific investigations. The protean character of mental illnesses was, of course, itself an obstacle, but I think this was exaggerated and mistaken for difficulties that lay in mankind's reactions to insanity rather than in the phenomena themselves. Neither insanity nor cure were adequately defined, and the fields of inquiry and action, in consequence, had no stable limits. What boundaries there were tended to shift about according to expediencies and changes in public feeling.

The lack of those indispensable conceptual tools – standard terms and definitions – encouraged the lumping together of phenomena that were widely different under the single term, "*insanity*." This usage, as noted in Chapter 2, led to lump thinking about what was actually heterogeneous, and thus inhibited the exercise of discrimination.

In such a climate, the specification of goals and the ordering of priorities was difficult. The effort of the mental hospital movement to cure every kind of illness with hospital environmental treatment was tantamount to striving for a large array of coequal goals that were not coequally feasible, in other words, the Lord Ronald syndrome. There was recognition that patients who had been ill less than a year had a better chance of recovery than those who had been disturbed for a longer period, but this observation does not seem to have served as a stimulus for efforts at systematic assessment of and discrimination among various types of disorders, or for an analysis of the implications of variations for care.

The mental hygiene movement

The origins of mental hygiene

The mental hygiene movement can be considered to have begun with the founding of the Connecticut Society for Mental Hygiene in 1908. There were, however, a number of historical trends that paved the way. We have already discussed one of these, concern about the worsening of conditions in public mental hospitals.

A second was the development of neurology as a subspecialty of medicine, with neurologists undertaking extensive private practices in the care of milder mental illnesses. This development was part and parcel of the widespread belief in biological determinism and was strongly encouraged by contemporary advances in knowledge concerning the structure and functioning of the brain. Interest in this had arisen in America from clinical studies of cranial injuries sustained during the Civil War and had been further encouraged by subsequent European research into cerebral localization. Virtually everyone believed that mental illnesses were due to brain disease, but, in contrast to mental hospital superintendents, the neurologists came to concentrate on the milder disturbances of emotion, feeling, and thought, which they considered to be manifestations of such physical disturbances in nerves as overexcitation, malnutrition, and exhaustion. It was in terms of these theories that Beard suggested the word *neurasthenia*. By 1880, numbers of neurologists were caring not only for what would today be accepted as neurological disorders but also for much of what would now be called psychoneuroses, or, in terms of DSM-III, or dysthymic, anxiety or dissociative disorders.

The neurologists, and their patients, believed that they were engaged in scientific practice, but, in fact, in this work they had no more scientific justification than did the proponents of moral treatment. *Neurasthenia* and other words referring to supposed physiological disturbances of the nerves became euphemisms by which to deny and sublimate the mental and emotional aspects of the disorders. As such, they were the forerunners of the use of *mental health* to mean, and yet at the same time to deny, mental illnesses.

The mental hospital superintendents, who were often still influenced by theories of moral treatment, claimed that adequate care could be given only in a mental hospital. This conviction, however, was not based on empirical evidence, because, as we have seen, clinical research in public mental hospitals had never amounted to much despite Pinel's example. Desire for scientific procedures, albeit in organic terms, lay with the neurologists, but when they endeavored to penetrate the hospitals, they were rejected by the superintendents.[35] Out of this situation arose one of the first of those ideological splits that, combined with competition for patients, have since done so much to undermine effective treatment for those with mental illnesses.

The sentiments of the neurologists toward the superintendents can be illustrated by two quotations. In 1879, Hammon[36] accused psychiatrists of diligently inculcating the idea that they alone, by education, by experience and by general aptitude are qualified [to care for mentally ill individuals] no matter what the type of mental aberration.'' Fifteen years later, Weir Mitchell,[37] speaking to a group of superintendents said, ''The cloistral lives you lead give rise, we think, to certain mental peculiarities . . . You hold to and teach certain opinions which we [i.e., neurologists] have long learned to lose. One is the superstition (almost is it that) to the effect that an asylum is in itself curative.''

In 1880, a number of neurologists and charity workers combined to form the National Association for the Protection of the Insane and Prevention of Insanity. Although this organization lasted only four years, it had a number of noteworthy attributes. First, it was dedicated to several familiar themes, namely humanitarian reform, the use of science, and the prevention of mental illnesses. Second, it incorporated the territorial dispute between the members of two different disciplines – neurologists and superintendents. Third, it came to reflect a serious difference between the physicians and the lay members. Both wanted reform, but, whereas the physicians thought reform should be based on scientific procedures and data, the laymen felt very strongly that they already knew what should be done and did not need to wait on such evidence. In the end, many of the neurologists came to the defense of the asylum superintendents against what they considered to be the blind emotions of some of the laymen. These differences in viewpoint were factors in shortening the life of the organization.

In addition to their participation in the association and in other ways helping to bring a scientific orientation into the public hospitals, the neurologists created an important model by their out-of-hospital care for the milder types of mental disorders. This helped set the stage for similar public services at a later date.

A third historical development leading to the mental hygiene movement was the establishment of "health centers" in some of the poor districts of cities to give free medical attention to those who could not afford private care. As neighborhood clinics, these centers established a precedent and demonstrated a pattern that mental hygiene clinics could later follow.

A fourth historical trend was the development of psychobiology at the turn of the century. This frame of reference included not only psychological and biological processes in the diagnosis and treatment of mental illnesses, but also familial, social, and cultural influences. It moved toward dissolving the neurologist–mental hospital polarities and toward placing the practice of psychiatry, both intramural and extramural, on a firmer clinical basis than had previously been the case. It is of interest, therefore, that the architect of psychobiology, Adolf Meyer, was not a member of either warring camp but a neuropathologist in a state hospital and, further, that he had come to the United States having been born and medically trained in a country well known for its ability to coordinate different cultural orientations and to remain out of destructive warfare, namely Switzerland. His influence was toward a constructive resolution of the conflict.

Becoming convinced in his pathology laboratory that biological determinism was a constricted view, Meyer extended his scrutiny to patient behavior, attitudes, life story, interpersonal relations, and social settings. In so doing, he synthesized, perhaps sometimes unwittingly, many ideas expounded by predecessors and contemporaries. These included, for example, not only Pinel and Tuke, but also Wundt, Wernicke, Jean-Marc Itard, Isaac Ray, John Minson Gait, John S. Butler, Kraepelin, Forel, Charcot, Bernheim, Janet, William James, John Dewey, and G. Stanley Hall.[38]

Psychobiology emphasized both the heterogeneity of mental illnesses and the multiplicity of causal factors and thereby restored social environment to a position of theoretical prominence. Meyer's feeling about biological determinism was similar to Coleridge's view of the eighteenth century mechanistic theory of the mind a hundred years before. Coleridge believed that the mechanistic theory was false, not because it did not tell the truth, but because it did not tell the whole truth.[39]

With psychobiology as his frame of reference, Meyer's struggle was to reduce reliance on speculative theory and to convert psychiatry into a field of scientific research and scientific practice[40] based on that research, by this means making it one of medicine's principal departments, comparable to internal medicine and surgery. He saw study of the personality and the interaction of social and biological factors as a necessary part of training in the preclinical years, more or less like anatomy and physiology, whereas the diagnosis and care of patients with mental illnesses should form a part of clinical training. To advance toward these goals, he developed a standard technique for examining psychiatric patients, a terminology, and a system for recording the facts of each case, together with methods for following the subsequent course of illness.

Professional recognition of Meyer increased after the turn of the century until he became the dominant influence in American psychiatry for a period of almost forty years. In 1913, he was appointed professor of psychiatry at Johns Hopkins University and first chief of the Phipps Clinic.

Because of its broad orientation, psychobiology opened the doors on ideas about prevention of mental illnesses. In postulating such multiple causes of mental illnesses as interpersonal experiences, habit formation, personal attitudes, and social environment, as well as biological factors, it raised the question of whether an individual could avoid some kinds of mental illnesses by avoiding the more noxious of these experiences and influences. In therapy, it seemed evident that much could be accomplished by changing behavior, attitudes, and, when possible, social situations. Might not such changes prevent recurrence? Might they not also prevent individuals from developing some illnesses in the first place? Meyer wrote and spoke a good deal about the importance of forming good "habits" and of developing helpful community agencies.[41] In so doing, he was covering much of the same ground that people do today when they speak of healthful life-styles and support systems.

The final trend to be noted has to do with *mental hygiene,* itself, as a concept and term. *Hygiene* was employed in the early part of the nineteenth century to mean the application of physiological knowledge to the promotion of health. In 1863, Isaac Ray defined mental hygiene as "the art of preserving the health of the mind against all the incidents and influences calculated to deteriorate its qualities, impair its energies, or derange its movements."[42]

The notion of hygiene became a part of the consciousness of educated people and has persisted until today. The concept of mental hygiene, however, appears to have faded until it was revived by Meyer at the beginning of the movement we are discussing and suggested by him as its name.

The Association for the Study and Prevention of Tuberculosis, founded in 1904, must have been an exemplar in the eyes of those concerned with mental illnesses. It stressed the relationship between disease and living conditions and "called for research into the social as well as the purely medical aspects of tuberculosis, popular education to prevent the disease, promotion of public and private sanitoria, and aid to indigent consumptives."[43]

Foundation and decline of the mental hygiene movement

The precipitating event in the formation of the mental hygiene movement was the meeting of Clifford Beers and Adolf Meyer in September 1907. Beers was a former mental patient who had written a book[44] about his experiences that was soon to become widely read and immensely influential. He wished to begin a movement that would bring about reform in mental hospitals. Meyer was impressed with Beer's abilities and sympathetic with this desire, being keenly aware of how bad the conditions were in many state hospitals and how easy it was even in the best of them for patient care to be mismanaged. But he also saw the desirability of going beyond this to community-based care, with emphases on the prevention of relapse and the strengthening of support systems. Looking back in 1930, he described his aims for mental hygiene as a

transformation of a relatively static attitude of mere mending into a vision and practice of more attention to the health, happiness, and efficiency of the rank and file of people – this is the turn from the charity and care and treatment in asylums and retreats to the spirit of hygiene, which is concerned with the problems and opportunities to keep well.[45]

Another prominent figure in the formation of the mental hygiene movement was William Alanson White, Superintendent of St. Elizabeth's Hospital in Washington, D.C. It was his view that

mental hygiene is therefore the last word in preventive medicine. The asylum, the prison, the poorhouse are where we find the results of failure. Such types of failure as are represented in these institutions will, of course, always be with us, but the work of mental hygiene is not primarily with them except insofar as they are salvable. Mental hygiene is primarily addressed to preventing such failures wherever possible.[46]

Meyer and White believed that a mental hygiene association would be a means of bringing together not only neurologists and hospital psychiatrists, but also general practitioners, members of other relevant disciplines, and influential lay people. They placed great emphasis on the association's members understanding and backing research and its application to policy, management, and practice. White said:

The mental hygiene movement has as one of its functions the encouragement of all those lines of inquiry and research that lead to a better knowledge of the human being, particularly of his conduct reactions. It is the task of mental hygiene to find less wasteful, more efficient means for dealing with the problems that arise at this level and, when found, to urge such measures unceasingly upon those who make and administer our laws and direct the trends of public thought.[47]

Meyer spoke of a "balance of forces . . . a mixture of humanitarian, fiscal and medical factors."[48]

Beers and Meyer established the Connecticut Society for Mental Hygiene in May 1908, and then, in February 1909, in New York, organized the National Committee for Mental Hygiene. It was a remarkably prestigious group composed of some of the most distinguished charitable workers, clergymen, and educators in the United States as well as leading psychiatrists and neurologists.[49] The Committee, however, was born without a working program because paralyzing differences in opinion were already manifest, differences that led to Meyer's resignation in 1910. In Sicherman's words,

Beers approached mental hygiene as a crusader and propagandist. He was naturally impatient with any delay in implementing programs which seemed to him only too necessary. He always hoped to secure a large endowment for the National Committee, and in his first proposal suggested that the organization act as a kind of "professional almoner" for mental hygiene activities.

Meyer hoped to avoid what he considered the propagandistic approach to mental hygiene. False claims and unrealistic expectations could only be followed by disillusionment, and a setback to progress in caring for the mentally ill. He urged Beers to establish concrete programs, such as after-care, rather than to concentrate on organizing state societies, collecting dues or distributing educational propaganda.

Meyer and Beers had established the Connecticut Society for Mental Hygiene in May 1908 as a pilot project to test the usefulness of mental hygiene work. Meyer did not wish to proceed nationally until the Connecticut Society had proven itself. He hoped it would implement concrete programs on a small scale, and considered after-care especially suitable for the purpose. For over a year he urged Beers, the executive secretary, to become involved in this work on a personal rather than an administrative level. He wanted Beers to assist ex-patients reestablish themselves, a task for which Beers must have seemed exceptionally qualified.[50]

William James summed up the differences as "a case of the ox and the wild ass." James also wrote in 1910 that Meyer's policy "would add piece to piece, and slowly widen from precedent to precedent, until by 1975 the whole country would rejoice in mental hygiene."[51] To one looking back from the present, these words appear less a gently sarcastic comment about Meyer than a regretful epitaph for the mental hygiene movement.

I have emphasized the differences between Beers and Meyer because they exemplify perduring issues that involved many people aside from the two of them. Moreover, despite the fact that the policies Beers advocated prevailed on the whole, struggles and turmoil continued within the organization. The four barriers described in Chapter 2 were plainly evident:

1   The heterogeneity of the field was not appreciated by many of the protagonists.
2   The emotions generated by the topic of mental illness tended to confuse most issues. As Meyer pointed out, "ignorance is strengthened by a natural feeling of awe and dread."
3   There was a failure to stick to scientific procedures and facts as a basis for action.
4   Too many goals and too few priorities continued to be articulated.

From its beginnings in 1908, the mental hygiene movement can be considered as having lasted some thirty years. It did a great deal in North America and around the world to awaken interest in the plight of mentally ill persons, especially in hospitals, and to promote concern about mental hygiene.

It also fostered the creation of numerous community mental hygiene clinics and gave major emphasis to the development of child guidance centers which were considered to be a means of preventing serious mental illnesses in later life. Child guidance, in fact, can be regarded as a movement in itself, and by 1928 there were 470 separate agencies serving children in the United States; by 1935, there were 617.[52]

Nevertheless, despite all these activities, the mental hygiene movement did not, as such, survive World War II. Enthusiasm had begun to wane some time before this, and many people began to wonder what was being accomplished. After all the years of effort, for example, there seemed to be only negligible changes in mental hospitals. Perhaps some improvements had been made in the 1920s, but these seemed to have been largely wiped out during the economic depression of the 1930s. Questions about the effectiveness of the community mental hygiene and child guidance clinics were not very satisfactorily answered. That they had been humane and given comfort to thousands of families was not to be doubted, but had they prevented anything? Had they improved "the health, happiness and efficiency of the rank and file of the people"?

Disillusionment mounted, and also fatigue with the topic. Some of this was no doubt due to larger shifts in public interests, but some was traceable to characteristics of the movement that have been sketched. It had neglected research on the results of its activities and had inspired expectations that were much higher than its ability to meet them. The effort by Meyer and White to establish a firm scientific foundation had turned out to be little more successful than that of Pinel at the beginning of moral treatment and the great mental hospital movement. As the mental hygiene movement grew, enthusiasms, emotional convictions, and ideologies came to the fore, and people began to practice more than they knew. Some of the later divisions in the movement were between those who wanted a commitment to eugenics and those who wanted a base in psychoanalytic theory.

Collective emotions, insufficiently restrained by disciplined thinking about facts, led to the resurgence of miraculous expectations. These swelled funding and membership but sentenced the movement to imprisonment behind the barriers.[53]

Mental hygiene in Nova Scotia

In comparison to the broader movement that has just been described, the mental hygiene movement in Nova Scotia neither rose so high nor fell so short of its expectations. Its origins went back to concerns about the poor, orphaned, and insane that, as we have seen, emerged almost as soon as the city of Halifax was founded in 1749. Aside from governmental measures and charitable work by churches, there were, in the nineteenth century, repeated efforts by private individuals and volunteer groups to help those who were destitute and handicapped to obtain food, shelter, clothing, fuel, and work. In the early years of the nineteenth century, associations of wealthy and influential men not only provided leadership in these matters but also did the actual visiting of poor families, analyzing their problems and supplying what was necessary.[54]

By the end of the nineteenth century, a major power in altruistic matters was the Halifax local of the Council of Women. One focus of their attention was the miserable state of the feebleminded. Retarded girls, in particular, were a topic of concern because they were subject to sexual abuses and were therefore likely to produce numbers of illegitimate retarded children. The council enlisted the cooperation of interested and influential men to form the Nova Scotia League for the Protection of the Feeble Minded in June 1908. In 1912, this organization stimulated the creation of fifty branch leagues throughout the province, but its activities declined during World War I.

The accidental explosion of a munitions ship in Halifax harbor in December 1917 killed about 2,000 people and destroyed a large part of the city in a manner almost predictive of Hiroshima. The consequences were severe for the survivors, many of whom were stripped of economic and social supports. Among these were the mentally retarded, and their plight led the Imperial Order of the Daughters of the Empire to create in 1918 a small home with accommodations for ten or twelve. It was headed by Dr. Eliza Brison, who may well have been the first psychiatrist in Nova Scotia outside the provincial hospital. The home disappeared after a few years because of lack of funds, but Brison went on to a distinguished career dedicated to the development and provision of services to mentally retarded persons in Nova Scotia and New Brunswick.

In 1918, under the influence of Beers and others, Canada's National Committee for Mental Hygiene was formed in Ottawa, and shortly afterward the Halifax local of the Council of Women created a mental hygiene committee. This played a part in 1920 in the revival and reorganization of the League for the Protection of the Feeble Minded and its renaming as the Nova Scotia Society for Mental Hygiene. The scope was enlarged at this time to include other types of mental abnormality.[55]

In 1924, the Reverend Samuel H. Prince, who had obtained a Ph.D. from Columbia University, became Professor of Economics and Sociology at King's College in Halifax. He was elected president of the Nova Scotia Society for Mental Hygiene in 1925 and for the next three decades was a leader among those concerned about the lot of retarded people and the abuses and neglect into which hospital care of mentally ill persons had descended. His efforts recall those of Hugh Bell seventy years before. As a result of Prince's work and that of his associates, a Royal Commission Concerning Mentally Deficient Persons in Nova Scotia was established with Prince as a member. The commission's report, published in 1927, recommended establishing "mental hygiene clinics," and creating the posts of provincial psychiatrist and provincial social worker. Mental hygiene education was urged, and both government and voluntary agencies were seen as cooperating "under the direction of the psychiatrist." A major recommendation was the addition of an active psychiatric treatment unit to the principal hospital in Halifax – the Victoria General.

Despite the obstacles created by the economic depression of the thirties and the outbreak of war in 1939, Prince and his group were able to see results from their efforts. The post of provincial psychiatrist was eventually created, and a training school for mental defectives was built in Truro. Moreover, by the early forties, the Maritime School of Social Work had been established with Prince as its first director.[56]

These successes came in spite of formidable inertia and some active resistance. For example, the staff of the Victoria General Hospital opposed the admission of "mental" cases of any kind. The head of the hospital (and later the minister of health) spoke for many of the doctors and nurses when he said that he "would have no crazy people here."[57]

On the other hand, Benge Atlee, professor of obstetrics and gynecology on the Dalhousie medical faculty, had ideas very similar to those of Prince and became a strong and active ally. The cooperation of the dean of the medical school was also secured, and then a grant was obtained from the Rockefeller Foundation providing for the establishment of a psychiatric clinic on the premises of Dalhousie University and for the training in London and at Johns Hopkins University of a psychiatrist who would take charge of it. The clinic opened in September 1941.[58]

In 1943, the government appointed a Commission on Provincial Development and Rehabilitation. Among its recommendations was the creation of a division of mental health services, and this was established in 1947 within the provincial department of Public Health.

The mental hygiene movement in Nova Scotia, with its pragmatic emphasis on tackling the problems of the most disturbed individuals first, differed from the movement in the United States in that it was little touched until much later by the theories of psychobiology or psychoanalysis. In some ways, this was an advantage. From both of these orientations, some mental illnesses were seen as largely based on personality processes that are common to everyone but in certain instances become malfunctional. This view can distract attention from the practical problems of serious mental illnesses because it opens the way to seductive preoccupation with the illumination mental illnesses can shed on normal life.

There can be no doubt that some mental illnesses are comprehensible, and usefully so, in terms of the malfunctioning of otherwise normal personality processes. What is not true is that unvalidated theories and speculations generated by those who treat mental illnesses are necessarily applicable to normal personality functioning – or to abnormal personality functioning, for that matter. Similarly, speculative theories about normal behavior, such as have been generated by anthropologists and sociologists, are not necessarily valid for cases of mental illness. Being both a clinician and a scientist, Meyer well knew the difference between psychobiology as an enormous frame of reference and as a very small body of actual knowledge. As a frame of reference, it pictured the person as a whole in relation to a total setting and stimulated lines of theory building and investigation. As a body of knowledge, it warned against taking action on the basis of unwarranted assumptions.

This distinction, however, has always been easily lost from view, and it was so lost in the mental hygiene movement. The effort to employ science to control Lord Ronald proved ineffective. Impelled by complex shared sentiments that rose as the mental hygiene movement rose, Lord Ronald rode through the fences of science as if they did not exist.

The mental health movement

In dealing with this movement, I shall sketch only its prehistory and first stage, and not, as with the two previous movements, attempt to outline its course and outcome. My reasons for this are, first, that the mental health movement is still going on and, second, that its beginning more or less coincides with the beginning of the service that is the focus of our case study. The subsequent history of the mental health movement will therefore be treated in Chapter 5, as part of the context of the case study.

The roots of the mental health movement

The movement has roots that go all the way back to moral treatment and beyond, but it has been particularly affected by a burgeoning of ideas that took place mostly in the second quarter of the twentieth century. As a point of departure, let us note that during the latter part of the nineteenth century and the early part of the twentieth, some discerning inroads were made into the lump thinking that characterized understanding of mental illnesses. The classification schemes that resulted have been much criticized since then for arbitrariness and rigidity, and for becoming ends in themselves rather than steps toward greater comprehension. Nevertheless, numbers of useful distinctions were made. Through the work of Kraepelin and then Bleuler, the syndromes of manic-depressive psychosis and schizophrenia were described. Blood and spinal-fluid tests for syphilis and the locating of spirochaetes in the brain separated paresis from other mental illnesses, and Goldberger's work set apart the dementia of pellagra.

These latter studies were, of course, major successes for the organic approach to insanity described earlier. Unfortunately, they contributed to the narrow view that biological factors are the only determinants of mental illness worth considering. This view encouraged inexpensive custody, as we have previously noted, but it also went beyond this, even to physical cruelties. For example, there was, for a time, a dogma maintaining that hidden foci of infection were the roots of mental illness.[59] The consequence of this was that innumerable patients were subjected to high colonic irrigations and to being deprived of tonsil and adenoidal tissues, appendixes, and all their teeth.

Psychobiology, which emerged amid these trends, has already been touched upon, but it is appropriate here to address some additional points. Meyer, in reaction against the doctrinaire character of existing nosologies, developed his own system for classifying psychiatric disorders based on patterns of behavior and expressions of feeling, developmental sequences, and evident degrees of disability.[60] In this effort, Meyer tried to do justice to the heterogeneity of psychiatric phenomena and especially to the variations among individuals, and he also tried to avoid what he considered the procrustean tendencies of other nomenclatures. He was, for instance, critical of diagnostic labels that embodied prediction of outcome, such as dementia praecox (precocious deterioration of the mind), because he thought such labels would be more than a psychiatrist could know at the time of diagnosis and were an unwarranted discouragement to effort on the part of therapist, patient, and family. He also felt that terms embodying purely theoretical assumptions, such as schizophrenia (split mind), should be avoided because they could lead to false conclusions about individual patients. Although recognizing the necessity of terms, he consistently warned against the danger of labels that overgeneralized and, thus, would inhibit discovering those assets and liabilities of each particular patient that could be employed in case management and treatment. He preferred to think of "reaction types" rather than disease entities and designed his terms and descriptive definitions so that they could be made to fit the actual facts of each patient's disturbance.

Although skeptical of "cures," Meyer was optimistic about improvements, recoveries, and restorations to useful and pleasurable living, and he believed that there were very few patients who could not be helped to some extent. Disorder was seen to a major degree (though not exclusively) as a product of past and current experiences; and opportunity for recovery was seen in terms of assets in both the patient and the environment that were not being sufficiently utilized. Treatment was seen as a matter of orchestrating these resources – physical, psychological, familial, social, and economic – toward better functioning, and of proceeding step by step during the treatment period to more adequate knowledge about the patient in all spheres of practical relevance, with suitable diagnostic reformulations from time to time. Meyer's conception of treatment may be summed up as a systematic personality study undertaken with the patient as an active partner in working toward his recovery.

The holism of psychobiology was very similar to that of Jan Smuts,[61] and, hence, it placed mental illness in a vast context of interacting forces. Meyer thought of these as organized in *"levels of integration."* Physical and chemical levels were thus seen to underlie the psychological level, and above this was a social level of integration.

In formulating psychobiology, Meyer was in contact with members of the Chicago school of sociology, particularly George Herbert Mead and W. I. Thomas. There was apparently considerable mutual influence. In later years, he was also in touch with such anthropologists as Bronislaw Malinowski, Ruth Benedict, Margaret Mead, and Clyde Kluckhohn.[62]

Meyer's interest in holistic theory was balanced by a pragmatic and empirical approach to the care of patients. He felt it was irresponsible to apply any but the best established theories in the treatment of ill people, and he was suspicious and critical of all schools and fashions in therapy, as well as of all dogma, unless they could show actual results. This distinction, however, was not always maintained by his followers, some of whom found in psychobiology more expansion of horizon and stimulus to speculation than they found a basis for definitions tied to observable phenomena and procedures of verification. They failed to make the distinction Meyer made between speculative theory, on the one hand, and patient care, on the other.

Psychoanalysis, although launched at the end of the nineteenth century, came into prominence after World War I and soon overshadowed psychobiology. It assumed the proportions of a movement, which psychobiology never was despite its impact on psychiatry, on medical education, and on some of the leaders in the social sciences. Consisting of both a new treatment technique and a highly original body of theory, psychoanalysis played a major part in the evolution of psychiatry as a specialty and in the growth of private practice beyond the level that had been reached by neurology. Psychoanalytic ideas also influenced the care of patients in hospitals, particularly private hospitals, and psychoanalysis supplied the theoretical underpinnings for psychosomatic medicine. Drawn into the field were numbers of people with brilliant minds and great capacities for teaching and leadership, including Adler, Jung, Jones, White, Sullivan, Alexander, Fromm, Horney, and the Menningers, to name but a few. The explanatory ideas and the procedures appealed strongly to numerous searching, educated, and financially well-off people in Europe and in North America, especially in the United States.

The influence of psychoanalysis, however, extended far beyond psychiatry and clinical psychology. Indeed, it reached into virtually every corner of the intellectual world. The impact was particularly strong in art and literature. Ever since the time of Flaubert and Baudelaire, artists and writers, turning away from romanticism, had been nibbling at the mores and self-confidence of the middle class, and they eventually mounted an all-out attack. In so doing, they drew heavily on psychoanalysis for ideas and symbols – the Dadaists provide an illustration.

Although in communist countries Marxian and Freudian theories have generally been considered incompatible, young radicals have nevertheless often drawn on psychoanalytic thought.[63] They have been attracted to the idea that the constraints imposed by society on instinctual development are a cause of mental abnormality, and they have used it in political philosophies that demand the destruction of authority systems and freedom for the individual.

Thus, one way and another, a great many people became more or less acquainted with psychoanalytic ideas. Even when information was oversimplified, distorted, and fragmentary, the sheer prevalence of psychoanalytic ideas helped create a feeling that they must contain some truth. This, in turn, facilitated application of the ideas in all sorts of mental hygiene programs aimed at the control and prevention of mental illnesses and at the development of more healthy personalities. Although there were opposing views, as for example from those with a strong biological orientation, and although there were a number of different schools of psychoanalytic thought, there was, nevertheless, enough confidence in basic validity of the ideas so that assertions of effectiveness were rarely put to the test.

Despite the difference in content, psychoanalysis had a number of characteristics in common with moral treatment and the mental hospital movement. Belief and enthusiasm far outran objective evidence. Expectations of results became exceedingly high, involving not only the cure of neurotic disorders but the alteration of fundamental psychic processes so that almost everybody might achieve new levels of competence, maturity, and self-realization. Though some proponents were modest in their claims, others leaned to omniscience, and their pronouncements encouraged overconfidence and overexpectation. In this, they resembled the omniscient mental hospital superintendents whom Weir Mitchell had criticized.

Like the moral treatment advocates, psychoanalysts tended to disregard the social consequences of the per patient cost of treatment. This meant that any hope of having an impact on the mental health of large populations – as in the child guidance movement – was in the long run stopped by the economic and personnel problems outlined as barrier four in Chapter 2.

Development of the traits of an ideology, such as emotional intensity and intolerance of dissent, was also a marked feature of psychoanalysis. This was encouraged by the fact that large numbers of both analysts and patients were convinced by their subjective experiences that the ideas and methods were valid. It was frequently said that one had to undergo psychoanalysis in order to understand its truth. Such a statement, of course, is not compatible with a scientific orientation, but it is characteristic of religions and cults.

Perhaps the most important comparison to be made between psychoanalysis and moral treatment and the mental hospital movement is in regard to scientific orientation. Psychoanalytic theory proved enormously stimulating to thought about human psychology, but the "metapsychological" emphasis distracted attention from the generation of hypotheses that could be tested with data. This is not to say that no good research was inspired by psychoanalysis. Obviously, some was; examples such as the studies of Sears, Bowlby, and Hilgard can be cited. Overall, however, the thrust was not in that direction. The emphasis was on the deductive application of theory (assumed to be true) to the interpretation of patients' feelings and behaviors. With this went comparatively little attention to the classification and measurement of more objectively accessible phenomena. Indeed, efforts to develop a systematic taxonomy were denigrated as largely useless and irrelevant, because it was the underlying symbolic meanings of symptoms, not their surface patterns, that mattered. Such observation and inductive thinking as was done generally stayed within boundaries set by the main tenets of the theory and rarely challenged them. Unfortunately, too, when challenges came from outside, they were apt to be, like the defenses, polemical. All in all, then, psychoanalysis was much stronger in creating theories and hypotheses than in verifying them.

A third major expansion of ideas about mental illnesses during the second quarter of the twentieth century came from the social sciences. This term includes several disciplines, but those that are most germane in this context are anthropology, sociology, and psychology, together with the intermediate social psychology. It is not possible, of course, to summarize all the relevant work of the social sciences in the space available here, but three topics may be selected as examples: culture, social organization, and stress.

The concept of *culture* embodies the fact that each generation passes on to the next not only its genes but also goods, property, language, customs, and shared sentiments about the nature of the world and the meaning of life. In addition to what can be inculcated and learned through conscious effort, culture is thought to include much that is acquired and retained at more or less unconscious levels. The culture of a society, in short, presents a "psychological reality"[64] that each member experiences from childhood to old age and that shapes each individual's personality.

As anthropological field studies from around the world succeeded in mapping an array of contrasting cultures, it became apparent that many of these "psychological realities" differed markedly from one culture to another. This led to the expectation that corresponding differences in personalities would also be found. Beyond this, it seemed likely that some of these culturally induced personality characteristics might lead to or actually be forms of mental illness.[65] Thus, the field of culture and personality became of major interest in the study of mental illnesses. A number of psychoanalysts and psychoanalytically oriented anthropologists were attracted to the field, and, through comparative studies, theories were developed to explain how adult personalities were determined by infant experiences. A notable example of collaborative effort was that of the psychoanalyst Kardiner and the anthropologist Linton in the late 1930s.[66] Generally, it came to be widely believed that populations with different cultures have different kinds and different frequencies of mental disorders and that, possibly, in some groups with psychologically benign cultures, there might be no disorders at all.

Two influential ideas came to the fore in this work: cultural determinism and cultural relativity. Cultural determinism views culture as the main, if not the only, cause of mental illness;[67] it has been advanced in opposition to biological determinism. This issue was and is of immense theoretical interest in efforts to explain the causes of both mental health and mental illnesses. Cultural relativity takes the view that all sentiments are relative to the culture in which they occur. What is right in one may be wrong in another, and vice versa. Polygamy is a crime in one group but approved in another; the same is true of homosexuality. All mental illnesses, in these terms, can be seen as behavior that is disfavored in Western culture but that may be accepted or even revered in others. People we call schizophrenic, for example, may be accepted as holy persons and mystics in parts of Asia. In its extreme form, cultural relativity raises the question of whether any such thing as mental illness actually exists, and even a moderate form would provoke serious questions about the manner in which we have been conceptualizing the phenomena we call mental illnesses and the ways in which we have been going about their control and prevention.

Social organization refers to the fact that cities, towns, and hamlets are divided into groups of people who work together for the survival of the whole. Thus, every human population cluster, no matter what its culture, is a system made up, or "organized," into subsystems, such as families and work units, interacting with one another. Within the subsystems, the basic unit of organization is conceived to be the *role*. Roles are filled by individual human beings, and the meaning of the term can be indicated by such words as husband, wife, father, mother, teacher, policeman, shopkeeper, minister, and so on. Every role includes sentiments and behaviors that the incumbent is expected to hold and perform.

George Herbert Mead, whom I have mentioned as an influence on

Meyer, developed a theory of personality based on the fact that every child grows up surrounded by people performing roles.[68] Mead suggested that children incorporate psychologically the roles of the persons with whom they interact, especially those who are of particular significance. Thus, in maturity, the individual's personality comes to be a synthesis of the roles that have been incorporated. This idea was responsible for a shift of emphasis not only from genetics but also from the infancy experiences that were the focus of psychoanalysis. It attached importance to the experiences of individuals at somewhat older ages and to the social environment outside as well as inside the family. Implicit in it was the thought that defective role models could produce deviant personalities, some of which would constitute forms of mental illness. Mead's thinking impressed Meyer as a systematic way of looking at the influences of environment on personality formation, and it played a part in the development of psychobiology. Others who followed Mead took up role theory and role study, and some pointed to society as a source of both mental illnesses and criminal deviances through the noxious organization of its roles and role relationships.

Adopting an ecological frame of reference from biology, a number of sociologists viewed society as an ecological system occupying a geographic area. In a classic work, Faris and Dunham[69] showed that there was a relationship between high admission rates of schizophrenics to hospitals and their residence in those ecological areas of Chicago that were marked by social disorganization and individual isolation. One result of this work was the formulation of two particularly important hypotheses: (1) that disorganized social environment causes schizophrenic disorders; (2) that people with schizophrenia drift into disorganized areas. As one might expect, social environmentalists favored the first hypothesis, whereas biological determinists were attracted to the second.

Contemporaneous with role and ecological research came investigation of social organization in terms of class levels. Holistic trends in both sociology and anthropology led to the study of total communities, such as towns and cities, and these invariably revealed marked stratification. W. Lloyd Warner's investigation of "Yankee City,"[70] conducted during the thirties, broke new ground in the understanding of North American towns. Warner and his co-workers defined and described six socioeconomic class levels and showed that sentiments, perceptions, and experiences of the people were different from one class level to another. Here again were implications for a variety of influences on personality formation and, through this, on mental illnesses and mental health. Of particular relevance was the concept of *anomie*. This concept had been developed earlier by the French sociologist Emile Durkheim in connection with his study of suicide, and it refers to a social condition in which values and norms are weak or nonexistent. The work on socioeconomic class in cities pointed strongly to the occurrence of anomie at the lower levels. Many people supposed that if anomie could lead to suicide, this was more or less the same thing as leading to mental illness.

The notion that psychological *stress* can disorder the mind was doubtless very old and widespread long before Shakespeare wrote about Ophelia. The "shell shock" experiences of soldiers during World War I and the miseries and suicides of the depression years of the 1930s helped to make the topic of scientific interest in this century. Some theory development occurred in both psychoanalysis and psychobiology, and experimentally based ideas were provided by Pavlov, Gantt, and Selye.

Stress theories also generated studies in both culture and social organization. For a time, there was a proliferation of work that attempted to compare cultures defined as tough and easy, continuous and discontinuous, competitive and cooperative, stable and rapidly changing, and so forth. Roles and role relationships in organizations were also studied and classified in terms of stress, and there emerged some evidence that certain roles were conducive to psychosomatic disorders such as peptic ulcer and hypertension. Also, the work on socioeconomic class structure suggested that people in low-income levels experienced a complex of exceedingly stressful conditions.

The Second World War brought forth new facts about stress. These are reported in the works of Grinker and Spiegel[71] and Lewis and Engle.[72] After observations made at the retreat from Dunkirk, there no longer seemed to be reason to doubt that severe environmental conditions could precipitate psychiatric disorders.[73] Neither genes nor childhood experiences were ruled out, of course, but they could be regarded as predisposing rather than as immediate causes. Environmental situations that produced stress thus took on renewed importance and raised questions as to whether the less drastic but nonetheless chronic and wearing stresses of peacetime civil life might not also play a causal role in some kinds of mental illnesses.

The other side of this was the possibility that certain kinds of environment might fortify personalities against the precipitation of psychiatric disorders in the face of stress. Numbers of writers on military psychiatry indicated that it was possible to create patterns of leadership and group attitudes such that later, under battle conditions, psychological casualties would be much reduced. With regard to therapy, it came to be recognized that better results were obtained if treatment were given immediately and geographically close to where the disturbance occurred and if the patient were returned quickly to his military unit.[74]

When these wartime experiences were reexamined in terms of peace and civilian life, they gave new impetus to theories of social and cultural causes and suggested the desirability of quick treatment, close to home, and with as little absence of the patient from roles in family and community as possible. Part of the thinking was that, insofar as immediate environmental stressors were a factor in the patient's illness, the treatment should enable him to find ways of coping and should avoid burdening him with the additional stressors of isolation in an institution and the difficulty of coming back as a partial stranger to his family and community. These ideas were a reawakening of earlier psychiatric thinking and were reinforced by numbers of trends in the social sciences that emphasized the psychologically supportive character of social groups and the psychological dependence of individuals on their culture.

There was, of course, awareness of the alternative situation in which the environmental stressors were beyond the individual's coping abilities. In this situation, there seemed to be the possibility of prevention through altering aspects of culture and social organization so as to reduce stressors and create more resources. Psychiatry thus came to be seen as having a public health dimension.

To the social sciences and psychiatry, as to other disciplines, the war brought problems that could not be answered by any one discipline alone. Collective thinking and cooperative action in problem solving reached proportions never previously seen, in such endeavors as the building of military morale, the selection of personnel for special duties, the analysis of Japanese morale, the military government of civilian populations, and the conduct of psychological warfare.[75] New methods for testing and screening individuals and for conducting surveys emerged; and the apparent practical success of some enterprises inspired high hope for their application in peacetime.

There was also, however, a negative side. Joint efforts among the disciplines sometimes led to a trading back and forth of terms and ideas that became distorted in passage. This interchange created a false sense of knowledge and familiarity across disciplines and contributed to endless confusions and passionate miscommunications in subsequent years. The need for a frame of reference grew rather than diminished, but interest in having one that bridged the disciplines soon declined after the war.

Although there was intellectual ferment among those involved in the diagnosis and treatment of mental illnesses, because of contact with the social sciences and the expansion of ideas this stimulated, clinical psychiatry as a whole was not at this time much affected. Diagnosis and treatment with orientations based on psychoanalytic theory were the dominant concerns of the vast majority of psychiatrists. Many were aware of the ferment, but more as casual spectators than participants. They were not persuaded that it had much to do with their daily concerns or with their futures. During the war, most psychiatrists had continued to perform the clinical work they had been trained to do, albeit, for many, in a military setting. After the war, they returned to or continued doing the same thing in civilian life. Despite the formation of the Group for the Advancement of Psychiatry and a progressive forward-looking thrust on the part of new leaders in the American Psychiatric Association, the overwhelming emphasis was on private services and the relevant knowledge and skills.

In the meantime, however, other trends were beginning to be perceptible. One of these was within the federal government of the United States, in which by the late 1930s the concept of a national psychiatric institute was already being discussed. World War II interrupted this development but gave impetus to the idea through experiences with "battle fatigue," efforts to increase combat morale, realization of the rapidly expanding need for postwar psychiatric rehabilitation, and the discovery that some 17 percent of American men were unfit for military service on psychiatric grounds. In 1944, Robert Felix, chief of the division of Mental Hygiene in the U.S. Public Health Service, presented to the public health surgeon general a proposal for a national mental health program. This led to the National Mental Health Act of 1946 and shortly thereafter to the founding of the National Institute of Mental Health. From this, there soon flowed enormous resources for programs, research, and education in "mental health."[76]

Mental hygiene and mental health

At this point, it is appropriate to pause for a moment to consider the origin and meaning of the term *mental health* itself, inasmuch as the development of the term is highly significant in the development of the movement. One reason for its selection may have been the location of the U.S. federal program in the Public Health Service, and *health* was part of the parent organization's name. The expression *public mental health,* though used, was perhaps too clumsy to survive. At any rate, what is salient is that one of the meanings of mental health is clearly in the public health tradition: the control and prevention of diseases. In this sense, health means the absence of disease.

Another influence that contributed to the use of the term with a different meaning was the further development of the division within the mental hygiene movement between those who were primarily illness oriented, consisting of some, but by no means all, of the physicians and nurses, and those who were health oriented, consisting of everyone else and comprising a much larger number. Writing as long ago as 1932, Adamson, a psychiatrist, said that the cleavage "must be eradicated before mental hygiene can come to its just fruition." She attributed the split to differences in education and training and pointed out that whereas medical personnel were grounded in an organic orientation, social workers "are educated in our general colleges and schools of social work where the emphasis of man has been placed on that subtle thing called 'mind' and only through academic psychology, philosophy, economics and sociology has he been explained."[77] The same could be said about many of the lay persons interested in mental hygiene.

By 1947, the issue was being described as a crisis. George Preston, a psychiatrist with long experience as a state commissioner, wrote:

Unless we meet this crisis and solve it, nonmedical persons with little knowledge of psychiatry will take over . . . In addition to the treatment of patients in hospitals, psychiatry today includes the treatment of habit disorders in well babies, of emotional disturbances and behavior disorders in children, of marital disorders, of impotence and frigidity, of gastric ulcers, of hypertension, of cardiac neuroses, of obsessional states, of phobias, of the whole realm of social maladjustments. Present day psychiatry touches obstetrics, gynecology, pediatrics, cardiology, surgery, internal medicine, and even dermatology.[78]

In this ideational and territorial struggle, *hygiene,* as a word, was seen to imply an organic orientation and medical domination. It could, of course, connote a team with psychologists and social workers as members, but the team would have a physician in charge. *Mental health,* on the other hand, implied personality development and the correction of bad environments, a field in which psychologists, social workers and others were fully qualified professionals in their own right. They saw in the abolition of the hygiene concept and label an opportunity for enhanced professional identity and greater freedom for decision and action.

Meanwhile, the National Mental Health Foundation had been established in 1946 by a group of former conscientious objectors who had been assigned to work in mental hospitals during the war. Horror-struck and angry over what they had seen, they felt that psychiatry as practiced in mental hospitals was wrong, and they questioned the validity of the whole psychiatric establishment. They considered the view of "mental illnesses" as illnesses to be simplistic. They also thought that the problems of prevention were far more complex than "brushing your teeth," a phrase they equated with the word *hygiene*.[79] It was society that needed to be renovated, not (as early mental hygienists had thought) the habits of individuals.

These views were congenial to the nonmedical mental hygiene workers and contributed to an amalgamation in 1950 of the National Association for Mental Hygiene and the National Mental Health Foundation to form the National Association for Mental Health. After this amalgamation, the term *mental hygiene* was less and less used, and *mental health* grew in popularity.

Another impetus to the change may have been a matter of public relations. In some ways, the National Association for Mental Health was a revitalization of the mental hygiene movement, and as such it had to show itself to be something new and different. A new name is a well-known device in such a situation.

Although there were common themes in the old and new movements, the differences were also genuine. Both focused on hospital reform, on community, on lay participation, and on prevention, but the mental health movement had much stronger nonmedical and antimedical components and went beyond the prevention of illness to the notion of vigorous, active promotion of health. The differences took shape in theory, ideology, and programming and encompassed many components whose relationships with one another were not well thought out.

Three common meanings of mental health exemplify the differences, inasmuch as each meaning is distinct from the others and two are antithetical. First, as we have seen, in the public health tradition the words mean programs, projects, and so forth, that are concerned with controlling and preventing mental illnesses. Mental health, in this sense, means the absence of illness and is not directly related to health promotion as such. Second, in the context of the National Association for Mental Health, mental health refers to ways and means whereby individuals can be happier, better balanced, more competent, and more self-realizing. Finally, in popular usage the words became a euphemism by which to escape from the unpleasantness of talking openly about mental illnesses. Having the same words mean both health and illness then led to coining the logically absurd term *positive mental health* in order to signal when *health* was not being used to mean illness.

The mental health movement in Nova Scotia

Events in Canada had many parallels to those in the United States, including an evolution within the federal government of concern about research and program development that resulted in the establishment of a major grant program in 1948. Although the same shift from mental hygiene to mental health took place, it did not reflect the influence of conscientious objectors or a very strong expression of feeling by nonmedical workers. The broadening of scope, however, was obvious, with some psychiatrists seeing their profession as covering the whole field of human well-being. Thus, Brock Chisholm, who became the first director general of the World Health Organization, defined *mental illness* as "any damage to the physical, mental or social functions of the human being resulting from his failure to adjust adequately to external forces of any kind, or to his own nature."[80]

In Nova Scotia, a sense of urgency about new goals was evident even before the war ended. In the report of the Nova Scotia Commission on Provincial Development and Rehabilitation in 1944, it was stated with regard to mental illnesses that

It should be possible gradually to transfer the emphasis of the total program from the purely institutional and treatment side, as it affects those who are already mentally ill, to the preventive and the clinical approach which concentrates on early diagnosis, early discovery of incipient cases and preventive treatment which is designed to cut down the need for later institutional care.[81]

The medical faculty at Dalhousie University in Halifax created a Department of Psychiatry with the aim of increasing the numbers of personnel available to meet the needs of the Maritime provinces. At the same time, the provincial government gave renewed attention to improving the quality of services in its institutions, to expanding their capacity, and to the creation of new services. In his 1947 report, the recently appointed chief of the Mental Health Administration[82] said, "an extended active treatment centre for all kinds of mental disorders, severe and mild, is being planned as an addition to the Nova Scotia Hospital . . . Prevention is constantly in our mind, along with providing the most modern and adequate facilities for diagnosis and treatment of existing disease." Toward the end of the report, he called for "more aggressive and persistent research."[83]

Concluding note

The year 1950 can be looked upon as a time of regrouping and resurgence in the mental illness field. Themes almost two centuries old intermingled with ideas generated by the experiences of the depression of the thirties and the war of the forties and by advances in the clinical and social sciences.

Belief in the power of psychological forces was in the foreground. Biology was not disregarded, but psychodynamics held the center of the stage. Personality was seen as shaped by events and by the ways the person perceived them. Intervention at a psychological level was thought to be effective, and there was a widespread return to confidence in the curability of mental illnesses. The problems ahead were seen as matters of learning more about how the psychological processes work and how to control them effectively.

There was renewed belief in the importance of environmental factors not only as causes of mental illnesses but also as opportunities for treatment and prevention. This was manifested in family treatment, group treatment, and therapeutic communities in which numerous echoes of moral treatment were perceptible. From war experiences, as well as from psychology and physiology, came awareness of environmental stressors. Anthropology and sociology introduced theories of cultural determinism, sociocultural change, noxious roles, socioeconomic class differentials, anomie, and social disorganization. The emergence of the applied social sciences raised the prospect of doing something about injurious environments so as to bring relief to people who were already mentally ill and to prevent others from becoming so. Expanded collaboration among the clinical and social science disciplines appeared to be essential, and the term *social psychiatry,* which had appeared in 1917 during the mental hygiene movement, once again came into prominence.[84]

Scientific research and the utilization of its results in scientific practice were seen as the obvious means for achieving rapid advances in the control and prevention of mental illnesses. The frontier for the advance was pictured by many of us as stretching across biology, psychiatry, psychology, anthropology, and the other social sciences. The emphasis on scientific underpinning was reminiscent of the hopes expressed by Meyer and White, at the beginning of the mental hygiene movement, and still earlier by Pinel, during the beginnings of moral treatment.

It was thought highly desirable that treatment be conducted as close as possible to where patients lived. This was partly a matter of bringing treatment to people who could not otherwise obtain it, an idea expressed previously, at the turn of the century in urban health centers and later in mental hygiene clinics. Involved also was the still older notion that prompt treatment could prevent the development of more serious conditions and reduce the necessity for hospitalization. To these beliefs, however, was added the weight of recent wartime demonstrations that immediate clinical intervention after a "breakdown" could restore a soldier to duty, whereas delayed treatment ran the risk of allowing chronic disorder to become established. Finally, there was a growing feeling that the ideal service would be one that focused on the population of a limited geographical area and thus allowed the staff to develop intimate knowledge of the people's needs, sentiments, and lifeways and to cultivate acquaintance among the population's leading physicians, teachers, and clergy. It seemed that such a realization would ensure a staff able to understand both patient needs and those resources of the local society that could be brought to their aid and also able to conduct mental health education in the manner best suited to the area. Underlying all these ideas was a fundamental humanitarian concern.

Perhaps the most important characteristic to note about the mental health movement, as it began to lift off in 1950, is the sense of excitement, pioneering, and imminent accomplishment that animated the participants. Psychodynamics and the social sciences seemed to be the keys to life. The interest of those who controlled political power and money seemed aroused as never before. Lawrence K. Frank expressed our feelings well when he said that we were at "the beginning of a self-conscious effort to reorient our culture and our social order in the light of the awareness, the insight, and the understandings now becoming available, to help us advance toward the human dignity which is both the prerequisite to, and the product of, mental health."[85]

We believed that almost every human being had a basic potential for that mental health, a potential that would assert itself if only given the opportunity.

4   The formation of a mental health center at mid-century

However much of a dreamer I may be, I pride myself on having seen a good many of my dreams come true. Can you see the ward or district organization with . . . a district center with reasonably accurate records of the facts needed for orderly work? Among the officers a district health officer, a district school committee and a district improvement and recreation committee . . . a tangible expression of what the district stands for?

I long to get the means and the privilege of trying a few mental hygiene districts, no doubt best shaped, as things are now subdivided, so as to have the school of the district as the center of attention, – with a specially trained physician and two or three helpers living in the district without any trumpets and without legislation; as far as possible inconspicuous, but charged to obtain the friendship and cooperation of the teachers . . . the district workers of various charity organizations and the physicians and ministers of the region. They would have to know their districts as a social fabric and they can do so if their districts are not too large; they must become helpers of individuals and families when they are in the mood to listen.

Adolf Meyer[1]

Founding the Bristol Mental Health Centre

The Bristol Mental Health Centre[2] grew out of the provincial government's plan (mentioned in Chapter 3) to establish care for all mentally ill persons throughout the province of Nova Scotia. Until that time, care for the chronically mentally ill in rural Nova Scotia had taken place mainly in municipal or county "hospitals." The quality of these institutions varied according to the humanity of the staffs and the degree of concern and financial resources of the municipal councils. Though some "hospitals" were kindly and decently managed, they were not suitable even for purely custodial purposes. Their budgets were too small, and the heterogeneous mixtures of human miseries and disabilities they contained were too great.

For acute illnesses such as depression and schizophrenic excitement,

53

the rural patient, like his urban counterpart, had access to the provincial hospital and, in later years, to a limited number of beds in one large general hospital and one veterans' hospital. The common route to the provincial hospital was through examination by local doctors and commitment papers, generally a measure of last resort. Technically competent, active treatment for the milder forms of mental illness, and for the early phases of the more severe kinds, was totally unavailable in rural areas. The vast majority of people with such troubles had to manage as well as they could – sometimes helped and sometimes rendered more disturbed by family, friends, and local practitioners who, at mid-century, had little or no training in psychiatry. For people who could afford them, the services of a few private psychiatrists were available, but only in the Halifax–Dartmouth metropolitan area.

The provincial government's idea of remedying the situation with a network of geographically dispersed clinics was both the cumulative result of work in Nova Scotia that extended back many decades and an expression of the national and international mental health movement. The province's effort was well in the van of many similar activities soon to get underway in other parts of North America.

From the beginning, however, there were problems in generating sufficient public interest and in securing personnel in adequate numbers. Although the provincial government's concern was shared by members of the mental hygiene association, by staffs in the social and public health agencies who recognized mental and emotional cases among their clients, and by numbers of physicians, there was no strong popular backing. Indeed, there were apt to be feelings of resentment and insult when it was suggested to people that their locality should have psychiatric services.

The personnel shortages were of the chronic type that had long plagued provincial and state hospitals. Given the size of its task (the province at that time had a population of about 642,600), there was also a severe shortage of staff in the headquarters of the provincial Mental Health Administration, where a single individual had to do virtually everything. In light of this dearth of staff, it is not surprising that attempts to create rural clinics ran into serious difficulties. By 1950, only one psychiatrist had been found who was willing to undertake such work, and he soon left for a more advantageous position.

At this point, coincidence played a facilitating role. My colleagues and I, as part of our projected Stirling County Study, wished to establish an outpatient clinic. It seemed to us that such a service would provide a means of helping mentally ill people located in the course of the epidemiological work, would be a practical return to the people of the area for their cooperation, and would yield case material integral to the research. When I brought these ideas to the province's Mental Health Administration, we were able to pool our interests and agree that a service would be established in Bristol, Stirling County's shire town. It was also agreed that the province would (with federal help) provide most of the funding for the Centre. Our research group, on the other hand, assumed responsibility for securing additional money from Canadian and United States sources, for recruiting staff, and for running the Centre, subject to the policies and regulations of the Mental Health Administration.

Funding for the Centre was then obtained from a number of sources. During the first six years, expenditures averaged $46,000 per year, about 57 percent of this coming from provincial and federal health grants and 43 percent from the Milbank Memorial Fund and the Carnegie Corporation of New York.

Patients were charged a token fee that varied according to ability to pay from twenty-five cents to five dollars per visit. Those who were really poor were generally not asked even for the twenty-five cents. The existence of this fee scale was a compromise between the government's policy of providing free service and disapproval of such a policy by the medical profession. The compromise was also supported by a belief among many psychiatrists that therapy worked better when patients paid and by the opinion of our local nonmedical advisors that many people would feel their dignity offended if no charge were made. The Centre's income from patient fees was never more than $1,000 per year, and after six years fees were abandoned.

The task of recruiting staff for the rural center proved troublesome for the Stirling County Study, much as it had for the provincial government. We were, however, able to supplement the small salaries dictated by the civil service regulations of the time. We were also able to give academic appointments to people in a variety of disciplines because the Study had the good fortune to be based in both the psychiatry and the sociology and anthropology departments at Cornell University. These and other advantages resulted in our securing two psychiatrists (one full-time and one part-time), a psychologist, a social worker, and a receptionist-secretary. The full-time psychiatrist was director of the Centre. It was planned that the members of the professional staff would divide their time about equally between research and service. To ensure that this would be feasible, the population served by the Centre was limited in the beginning to the approximately 20,000 people of Stirling County.

Meanwhile, we had been in touch with the growing number of practicing psychiatrists in Nova Scotia, with the Department of Psychiatry at

Dalhousie University, and with the provincial medical association, informing them about and seeking their goodwill and cooperation in the work. In Stirling County, parallel steps were taken to gain acquaintance with and to inform all the leaders and opinion makers throughout the area. This resulted in the medical association in Bristol becoming the formal sponsor of the Centre.

The end of the preliminary planning was marked by a ceremonial dinner in Halifax on October 21, 1950, attended by the president of Dalhousie University and the deputy minister of health. Also present were members of Dalhousie's Department of Psychiatry, the province's Mental Health Administration, some faculty from Acadia University, the newly appointed psychiatric staff of the Centre, and other members of the Stirling County Study. The following spring, the doctors in Bristol held a reception for the Centre staff and the Centre opened its doors to patients on June 1, 1951.

The number of new patients seen in a year averaged 160, but there was considerable annual variation, from 64 to 236, partly the result of changes in the boundaries of the geographic area for which the Centre was responsible. When these became stabilized after ten years to encompass a population of about 38,000 (following a period when there had been responsibility for a population of 80,000), the annual average of new patients became 177, with a range from 108 to 220. The vast majority of these were outpatients or those seen on home visits. The Centre, having no beds of its own, referred most of those requiring hospitalization to one of the hospitals in the Halifax area. A few patients were admitted from time to time for brief periods to the Bristol General Hospital.

The different kinds of mental illnesses seen are indicated in Table 1. The percentage of different disorders, in contrast to the variation in total admission rates, shows a high degree of consistency. This consistency is apparent over many changes in the Centre and the region during fifteen years and can be interpreted to mean that the interaction of the Centre and the population revolved around a fairly stable set of clinical problems.

Analysis of age and sex shows that young women suffering from anxiety and depression mixed with physiological disturbances – that is, psychoneurosis in pre-DSM-III terms – constituted the largest single category and the major part of the total case load. The female–male ratios among persons with this kind of disorder were 2:1 (1952) and 4:1 (1967). Furthermore, most of the women who sought help for the first time were married, which implies that aid from the Centre was important to families as well as to individuals.

The next largest group of patients consisted of people suffering from

Table 1. *Primary diagnosis of new admission adult patients seen in calendar years 1952 and 1967*

	1952		1967	
	Number	Percentage	Number	Percentage
Psychosis	18	21	15	23
Psychoneurosis	42	48	26	41
Personality disorder	11	13	6	9
Brain syndrome	9	10	8	13
Other"	7	8	9	14
Total	87	100	64	100

Note: Because of changes occurring in catchment area boundaries and because patients were often seen from outside the catchment area, this comparison is based on only those patients admitted from the study area where the boundaries remained constant.
"In 1952, these were 3 psychophysiological, 2 mental deficiency, 1 sociopathic, and 1 not ill. In 1967, these were 1 psychophysiological, 2 mental deficiency, 2 sociopathic, 3 not ill, and 1 no diagnosis.

psychoses, with these conditions belonging mainly in one of the schizophrenic-spectrum categories. Here again, there were more women than men, but there was far less discrepancy in their relative numbers. Nor were the first admissions for psychosis so strongly weighted with younger people.

Personality disorders were the next largest group. It also contained more females than males, and there was some tendency for the first admissions to be young.

Although brain syndromes occurred at all ages, most of those presented to the Centre were the type characteristic of later life. In 1967, there were again somewhat more women in this group, perhaps because of their tendency to live longer.

Goals

Starting in 1950, and building on the aims of the Mental Health Administration, the goals of the Centre were formulated before and during its founding and were a product of the Stirling County Study, including, of course, the staff of the Centre. The initial ideas were further developed and modified at meetings of the group held for that purpose in the autumn of 1953. These final goals were an attempt to translate into action the ideals and ideas summed up in the concluding note of Chapter 3. A short descriptive outline follows.

Diagnosis and treatment

A primary goal of the Bristol Mental Health Centre was to provide diagnostic and treatment services to a small town and the surrounding rural area. Diagnosis included a mental-status examination, medical, social, and psychological histories, and a synthesis of this information into a formulation of the patient's problems. Such a formulation was then to be the basis of case management, which could include psychotherapy, administration of the supportive medications available at the time (for instance barbiturates), counseling of patient and family members, and help with practical arrangements in the patient's residential or working relationships in such a way as to facilitate recovery. The maintaining of clear and detailed patient records on diagnosis, treatment plans and clinical course was considered essential for adequate service. It was anticipated not only that the same patients would return from time to time through the years, but also that other members of their families would come as patients and that the same family and community situations would likely reemerge as major factors in both illness and recovery. We believed that records would provide cumulative knowledge and that this was a necessary condition for providing quality care to people of the area.

A subsidiary goal was to maximize the effectiveness of the Centre by admitting patients at the earliest possible stage of illness. The expectation was that through early intervention more serious and chronic problems would be avoided and the whole disturbance of the patient's life would be shortened. We also thought it important to follow up patients returning from mental hospitals, because there would be in this aftercare an opportunity to detect recurrence of disorder at an early phase and, by prompt attention, to prevent rehospitalization. Home visits, in particular, were to be given high priority, again with the idea that prompt intervention in an early, acute phase of illness, and in the patient's own setting, would reduce both duration and severity of disturbance. (It was at this time that the work of Querido[3] was gaining attention.)

A second subsidiary goal was to expand services in the following ways:

> To increase the size of the population served – that is, to enlarge the catchment area
> To increase the proportion of people in the catchment area served
> To increase the varieties of services offered.

Developing a greater variety of services would, we believed, mean more effective treatment for more kinds of patients. We had in mind subcoma insulin therapy, electroshock, narcotherapy, hypnosis, group psychotherapy, family counseling, home-visiting services, diagnostic and treatment services for children, and the use of the general hospital for patients who were manageable in that environment – people with conditions such as acute anxiety or delirium tremens.

Consultation and referral

A second major goal of the Mental Health Centre was to offer consultation and referral services to other agencies in the geographic area, for example, the medical, school, welfare, religious, and legal subsystems of the larger society.

The medical subsystem. In addition to receiving patients referred by physicians within the area, it was expected that the Centre would refer selected patients back to their doctors for care. The intent was to have the physicians conduct the actual treatment of these cases in consultation with the Centre, and it was believed that in this way the impact of the Centre on the population would be multiplied. It was also thought that the doctors might consult the Centre psychiatrists regarding some patients whom the psychiatrists would not actually see. In other words, the Centre was to be a resource to which the physicians could turn for information and advice while themselves caring for patients with such disorders as anxiety and not very severe depression.

In addition to working with physicians, we hoped that the Centre would be able to counsel and train the nurses of the hospital in understanding mental health and illness and in caring for all patients, regardless of diagnosis, that were in an emotionally disturbed condition. The Centre was to give similar help to the public health nurses and the Victorian Order of Nurses (a privately supported group) so that they could more effectively demonstrate to families the home care of patients suffering from such disorders as chronic depression and senility as well as the care of the emotional components in organic illnesses. Finally, we hoped that the home-visiting nurses' alertness to the presence of psychiatric disorders would increase and that they would acquire an improved grasp of when it was appropriate to refer someone to the Centre.

The school subsystem. Improving the lot of children with psychological difficulties was, to our minds, of major importance; it also figured in our goal of the early diagnosis and treatment of mental illnesses. The Centre was to create a working arrangement with school teachers, counselors, and administrators whereby it could educate them regarding mental illnesses and mental health. Informal personal contacts, conferences, and seminars were to be encouraged.

The social service subsystem. It was planned that the Centre would collaborate with the province's social services through cross-referral and cross-consultation on appropriate cases. We also expected that the Centre would help social service personnel improve their clinical perceptiveness in dealing with their clients.

The religious subsystem. The Centre staff was also to establish mutual collaboration with the clergy. Information was to be offered regarding the resources of the Centre and mental illnesses more generally so that the clergy themselves could become more competent in working with troubled parishioners, especially those in the early stages of mental illnesses, and would know when to refer them to the Centre. It was also hoped that they would work with the Centre as aides in home visiting.

The legal subsystem. The Centre's goal in this area was not very extensive. It was prepared to offer technical advice to lawyers and the courts on request.

Research and evaluation

Research of a pragmatic kind, to be conducted by the staff, was a major goal. It was hoped that the treatment and prevention of psychiatric disorder in a rural setting could be illuminated through use of the following methods: developing a model; conducting an epidemiological survey to determine the actual prevalence of mental illnesses in the geographic area; and analyzing clinical cases in order to understand the local conditions and characteristics of mental illnesses.

A model for rural mental health centers. The provision of services for mentally ill persons in a small town and rural area was, to a large extent, unknown territory at the time the Centre began. Part of the Centre's mission, therefore, was to act as a forerunner for other rural mental health centers in Canada and the United States. It was intended that the Centre would collect basic information and explore a variety of such questions as the following: What kinds of illnesses and related personal problems occur most frequently? What kinds of treatments can be offered in a rural setting that will be of help with the commonly occurring illnesses? Can local resources be developed to increase the effectiveness of patient care? What organizational pattern would best suit area needs – for example, should there be satellite clinics in outlying districts with visits by a circuit-riding psychiatrist? How might forms of prevention be added to ongoing treatment modalities? How can individuals and organizations of the local area participate in the guidance of a mental health center?

Epidemiological survey. The Centre was to be the site of that part of the epidemiological research concerned with ascertaining the true prevalence of mental illnesses in the geographic area (the "dependent variable"). Although this work was heuristic, it was also meant to enable the Centre to understand, diagnose, treat, and refer patients more effectively. It was to be a foundation for outreach and prevention projects and was to guide the development of the Centre as a model for rural services.

Case studies. The third research aim was the long-term, intensive, and systematic study of cases coming to the Centre in order to understand better the characteristics of mental illnesses in this particular area. The results, we thought, would be of practical benefit in helping the Centre diagnose, treat, refer, and consult more effectively and, hence, would also contribute to the development of the Centre as a model for the care of rural mental illnesses.

Prevention

Primary prevention. The effort in primary prevention was to involve public education regarding mental health and illness so that people might cope better with putative causal factors such as psychological stress and mobilize their personal and social assets effectively. Specific targets were to be parents, teachers, physicians, clergy, people with political influence, and other leaders, opinion setters, and "gatekeepers" of society.

Secondary prevention. This was to consist of early treatment designed to prevent more serious illness, as already noted under the diagnostic and treatment goals.

Tertiary prevention. The goal here was to reduce disability in those who suffered from one of the chronic mental illnesses. Implementation was visualized in terms of maintaining chronically ill people at work and in active relationships with their families and the rest of the social environment, thereby drawing on whatever assets such individuals had and avoiding deterioration of capacities as a secondary consequence of illness. The social worker, in particular, was to orchestrate local resources – jobs, church, recreation, friends, family members – for keeping patients as active as their conditions would permit. It was hoped that the Centre could play a therapeutic and supporting role for patients without disrupting their places in the social network and local support systems.

Also included as a goal was making hospitalization in a mental institution unnecessary. We thought that maintaining the patient out of hospital would avoid family and community adaptation to his absence, which could render it difficult later for them to readjust their social equilibrium and readmit him to the group.

Development of area resources

Because small towns and rural areas lack many of the formal services available in a city, an important goal was to develop relevant resources in the geographic area. Our desire to find multiplier effects has already been mentioned in connection with referral and consultation, and public education has been mentioned under prevention. The notion of developing the area's resources carried these ideas further.

Our premise was that towns and villages as social systems are engaged in carrying out activities upon which their survival and well-being depend. In cities, many of these activities are formalized by the creation of special organizations and the promulgation of regulations. In less densely populated areas, these functions are often accomplished informally. That is to say, they are managed as problems to be solved according to unwritten customs within the framework of such general institutions as the family, the neighborhood, and the church. Welfare problems, for instance, were often handled this way in areas that lacked formal welfare programs.

Given this premise, the Centre's goal became twofold. One part was to discover family and neighborhood resources and to develop methods for utilizing them in conjunction with the Centre in order to aid patients more effectively. The second part was to identify and develop the help-giving potential of the formal organizations. Underlying this goal was our observation that in towns and villages some functional needs were met by people in formal roles undertaking more tasks than those indicated by their formal role titles. Thus, doctors, nurses, clergy, lawyers, and teachers often acted as counselors in psychological and human-relations problems.

And some employers, on their own, hired handicapped persons and tried to organize work so that it was within the capabilities of these individuals.

The utilization of research results

A major goal was to have the Centre make use of the research results obtained in the geographic area studied. Obviously, such a goal could only be stated in general terms until the research, itself, was done.

Training

The training of professionals in social and community psychiatry was highly valued by most of those who founded the Centre. We thought that the Centre ought to serve as a place where experience in rural and small-town work could be obtained by psychiatrists, psychologists, nurses, and social workers, and by students in these or related disciplines. The intention was to arrange for academic and professional credit.

Three kinds of training were visualized: (1) providing in-service experience for young staff members who came to work at the Centre for two or three years; (2) offering formal training to fellows, residents, medical students, nurses, social workers, and psychologists who spent a few months to a year at the Centre; and (3) conducting short workshops for still other professionals such as clergy and teachers.

Collaboration with universities

Academic collaboration occupied a high position among our goals. This was because we believed that such connections would do much to facilitate the recruiting and maintenance of well-qualified staff and, by this means, enhance the accomplishment of most other goals.

Outcomes

As part of our case study, data pertaining to the outcomes for each of the goals were scrutinized at length. The main conclusions may be summarized as follows.

Diagnosis and treatment

The provision of diagnosis and treatment for patients close to home was the best achieved and most steadily maintained of all the Centre's original goals. The Centre, once begun, never stopped providing these services during the years under review. This is not an insignificant achievement considering the four barriers discussed in Chapter 2, and it suggests that there was a vein of determination among professionals, people in government, and members of society more generally to do something for individuals with mental illnesses. At the same time, as we shall see later, single-mindedness about keeping the Centre open had its disadvantageous side.

As far as psychopharmacological treatments were concerned, these changed appropriately as scientific advances made more and more effective medications available for both mild and severe forms of disorders. This progress was aided by the evolution of governmental provisions for supplying drugs to those who could not afford them.

The size of the catchment area for the Centre also expanded, as was noted earlier in this chapter. The population serviced by the Centre jumped from 20,000 to 80,000 before stabilizing at about 38,000. On the other hand, there was no substantial increase over the years in the proportion of the population reached.

A decline in the quality of diagnosis and treatment took place after the first few years, and this was ultimately followed by a quantitative decline. The latter is evident in tabulations showing the numbers of patients being seen in a unit of time and in the numbers of minutes devoted to each.

The variety of treatments offered over the period of our case study was considerable, but their effectiveness was vitiated by the fact that very few were available simultaneously, so that what might have been a strength was actually a weakness. For example, at the time when a staff member was recruited who had some training in the problems of reading disabilities, there was not a psychologist at the Centre with training in psychological testing, counseling, or psychotherapy.

Furthermore, some of the services offered were uncontrolled experiments by staff members using techniques they had read about but in which they had not been trained. Janov's primal scream therapy is one example; this treatment, of course, is at best controversial, but in the instance in question it was indefensible because the individual practicing it had not had the training Janov himself insists is necessary.

The dispensing of drugs came to be characterized by a similar lack of control and by the exposure of patients to decisions on the part of staff members who were not qualified to make them. Medication renewals, for instance, were performed by secretaries without patients being seen by a psychiatrist or a nurse; some of these renewals were even done by correspondence.

The clinical record keeping, despite an adequate supply of dictaphones and secretaries, became little more than brief handwritten notes, generally lacking in clinical description, diagnosis, treatment plan, and sometimes even dates. From 1956 onward, there were many patient folders that contained no clinical information of any kind.

After some early utilization of the facilities of the local general hospital, the Centre moved progressively toward separating itself from that institution. Staff members said that patients could be treated better at home, that occupational therapy was lacking in the hospital, and that there were no rooms suitable for consultation. Only for the first of these was there a supportable argument, and that only in regard to some patients.

During the first years of the Centre's existence, comments from the general practitioners of the area were numerous and favorable. Gradually, however, negative criticisms grew in volume, and at the same time the psychiatrists at the Centre began to withdraw from the area's medical association. The physicians' criticisms included lack of attention to patients with suicidal depressions and psychotic disturbances, nonresponsiveness to referral requests, and failures of communication regarding medications. The last was important in order to prevent patients who were being seen by both the Centre and family physicians from accidentally receiving overdoses or incompatible combinations of medications. The criticisms were much discussed among the doctors and were communicated to the director of the Centre, but without, so the doctors said, any reduction in the problems.

In short, then, although in general terms the goals of establishing and maintaining a diagnostic and treatment service close to people's homes and of expanding the catchment area were achieved, the quality and quantity of treatment given did not meet expectations; nor were the variety of services offered expanded according to plan. With regard to the provision of early treatment and its effectiveness, no data are currently available by which this can be judged.

Consultation and referral

The goals of consultation and referral evolved along lines very similar to those just outlined for diagnosis and treatment. After a period of growing cooperation with the medical subsystem, there was a reversal of this trend and a breaking away by the Centre. This occurred despite the fact that, as shown in Table 2, most of the Centre's patients came as referrals from the doctors. In time, most of the general practitioners began to assert that they had discontinued referring patients to the Centre and that they pre-

Table 2. *Sources of referral for first admissions of adult patients in calendar years 1952 and 1967 (see note on Table 1)*

	1952		1967	
	Number	Percentage	Number	Percentage
Self	3	3.4	5	7.8
Family	2	2.3	7	10.9
Friend	0	0	1	1.6
Provincial hospital	2	2.3	3	4.7
Physician	77	88.5	40	62.5
Nurse	1	1.1	0	0
Clergy	0	0	1	1.6
Court and police	0	0	1	1.6
Welfare	2	2.3	5	7.8
Other	0	0	1	1.6
Total	87	99.9	64	100.1

ferred, instead, to treat those they could themselves and to use resources outside the area for the more serious cases. The latter course of action was, obviously, contrary to the goal of effective treatment close to home.

Consultation with and referral from the schools was also troubled. It started badly, improved at times, and then, in the case of certain schools, became an openly hostile relationship, culminating in public attacks by Centre personnel on the school authorities.

Consultation with and referral from the local agency of the province's social services developed satisfactorily. Although it fluctuated somewhat, this relationship came close to achieving the original expectations. On the other hand, not many patients were referred to the Centre from this source, and the relationship did not develop as a means whereby the Centre could increase its outreach to economically disadvantaged people.

With regard to the religious subsystem, progress was again up and down. Shortly after the Centre opened, the staff prepared a list of clergy and the areas they served. Many of these men were then seen and their assistance sought in case finding. Initially, this effort was part of the research, but it soon became a "coffee and conversation" group and ultimately a formal "clinical–clergy association." Fairly regular meetings were held, and films were often used to introduce topics for discussion such as "feelings of hostility," "only boy," or "feelings of depression." At times, a clergyman or staff member presented information relating to a common concern: normal and abnormal grief reactions, delinquency, psychiatric convalescence and rehabilitation, premarital counseling, marriage counseling, and so on. Of course, only a few of all the area's clergy joined in these meetings, geographic distance among other factors placing limits on who could attend. Nevertheless, there came to be a good working relationship whereby the Centre was able to get help from the clergy in the care of particular cases and the clergy could secure advice from the Centre regarding problems among their parishioners. The number of cases actually referred to the Centre by the clergy, however, was never large.

During the late fifties and through the middle sixties, meetings with the clergy went through several phases of changes and then decreased considerably in number. In 1967, the Centre sponsored a two-day institute on pastoral counseling with special reference to rural areas. Following this, formal activities virtually stopped, although meetings between particular staff members and particular clergymen continued from time to time.

One may summarize the outcome of consultations and referrals by saying that there was a great deal of activity and effort, that many projects were started but in most cases they failed to achieve stability, and that in some cases relationships with the Centre turned from positive to negative.

Research and evaluation

If diagnosis and treatment were the best achieved goals of the Centre, research was the worst achieved. Many data were gathered, but comparatively few of them were brought together in final synthesis and reporting by Centre staff. No written description of the model for a rural clinic was ever published, although it is possible that work done toward that end had helpful consequences for the Centre. After more than a year of floundering, the epidemiological research had to be removed by me from the Centre's jurisdiction and transferred to a separate unit set up specifically for that purpose within the Stirling County Study.

The goal of making case studies of Centre patients was actively pursued during the first five years and then allowed to lapse. Its pursuit resulted in one published paper.[4]

Prevention

As noted previously, the Centre's original goal in primary prevention was limited to public education. This was pursued with vigor for many years, although with what effect it is impossible to say.

In early 1970, the Centre staff members expanded the prevention goal to include a major thrust aimed at altering the social environment in Bristol. This grew out of the conviction that the schools of Bristol constituted a psychologically damaging environment for children. The methods employed included public accusation and confrontation together with demands for the ouster of school personnel. Staff members also helped precipitate a social crisis in Bristol that grew to considerable proportions (see Chapter 5). Among the consequences of this crisis for the Centre was a crop of negative opinions and attitudes on the part of the public and a certain amount of isolation from the other subsystems of the area, especially the human service organizations.

Other goals

There were some sporadic efforts and a few successes in the early years with regard to the development of area resources. For instance, some volunteer assistance was obtained in making home visits to isolated depressed patients. The main achievement, however, was that of helping to create a Board of Directors for the Centre in 1956. Composed mainly of local people, the Board had a complex influence on the subsequent functioning of the Centre which will be described in later chapters.

The utilization of research results derived from the Centre was, obviously, not very successful given that the Centre completed so little research. The research completed by psychologists, sociologists, and anthropologists in other units of the Stirling County Study might have been utilized in various ways by the Centre staff, but was not.

The training of professional personnel at the Centre did take place, but it could not be said to have flourished after the first five or six years. A few people received some academic credit for time spent at the Centre, but it was never possible to work out a regular program with a Canadian training center in any of the relevant professional disciplines.

Collaboration with universities was also only partially successful. Ties consisting of formal appointments, participation in seminars, and opportunities for staff professional development existed exclusively through the Stirling County Study. In the beginning, this meant the involvement of Cornell University, including both the Department of Psychiatry in the Medical School and the Department of Sociology and Anthropology in the College of Arts and Sciences. This involvement shifted to Harvard in 1966 when the Stirling County Study moved its base to the Department of Behavioral Sciences at the Harvard School of Public Health. Throughout this period there were cooperative relationships and many informal exchanges with Acadia and Dalhousie Universities in Nova Scotia. It had been my hope that there would be a gradual transition in which the link between Harvard and the Centre would eventually be replaced by a link to Dalhousie. The tie with Harvard was attenuated in the late sixties and broken in 1970, but no connection with Dalhousie took its place.

Concluding note

The discrepancies between goals and outcomes naturally raise the question of why these discrepancies occurred. Part of the answer has already been anticipated in the description, in Chapter 2, of the barriers that are intrinsic to the study, prevention, and treatment of mental illnesses. Other parts of the answer lie in broader social (extrinsic) factors. Both parts have been touched on in Chapter 3. The task now is to show more specifically the factors that did affect the operation of the Centre and the ways in which they did so. Before doing that, however, it would be useful to take a look at the historical and social context of the case study with particular attention to changes taking place in regard to both the intrinsic and the extrinsic factors that affected the mental illness field.

5 Another glance at history: relevant events in the century's third quarter

The slowing progress toward the Centre's original goals, and the abandonment of some, can be explained by characteristics of the goals themselves, the Centre, its Board of Directors, the Mental Health Administration, and the local society. All of these, however, were, in turn, directly and indirectly affected by more general social processes. We can begin, therefore, by looking at trends in the larger social matrix. This means continuing our glance at history from the point we left it in Chapter 3, that is, 1950, through the third quarter of the present century.

Progress and problems in the mental health movement

The optimism and forward thinking of the mental health movement in the early fifties was sustained over a period of years, as the following landmark dates indicate.

1954   Appointment of the Royal Commission on the Law Relating to Mental Illness and Mental Deficiency in the United Kingdom.

1955   Formation of the Joint Commission on Mental Illness and Health in the United States.

1957   Report of the Royal Commission on the Law Relating to Mental Illness and Mental Deficiency. It recommended putting mentally ill people on the same footing as patients with other forms of illness, admitting them to general hospitals, and expanding community services.[1]

1959   Passage of the British Mental Health Act, based on the report of the Royal Commission.

1961   Publication of *Action for Mental Health* by the Joint Commission on Mental Illness and Health in the United States. It recommended "a full-time mental health clinic available to each 50,000 of population" that would serve (1) "to provide treatment by a basic mental health team . . . for persons with acute mental illness," (2) "to care for incompletely recovered mental patients either short of admission to a hospital, or following discharge from the hospital," and (3) "to pro-

70

vide a headquarters base for mental health consultants working with mental health counselors."[2]

1963 Publication of *More for the Mind* by the Canadian Mental Health Association. This recommended that "psychiatric treatment services be established in centres of population on a regional basis" and that "mentally ill patients should be treated in local hospitals or clinics . . . as early as possible, with as little dislocation and as much continuity and social restoration as possible."[3]

1963 Signing into law in the United States of the Community Mental Health Centers Act. As summarized by President Kennedy, this was

> a national mental health program to assist in the inauguration of a wholly new emphasis and approach to care for the mentally ill. This approach relies primarily upon the new knowledge and the new drugs acquired and developed in recent years which make it possible for most of the mentally ill to be successfully and quickly treated in their communities and returned to a useful place in society.[4]

It is of interest to observe that as of 1963 Nova Scotia had established nine of its ten projected community mental health clinics. The Nova Scotia experience, therefore, can be looked upon as a precursor of what was to occur later in other areas.

Associated with the landmark events just noted were new discoveries in medication, as mentioned in the Kennedy statement. From their original adjunctive role, drugs moved to the center of the field in controlling the disabilities of schizophrenia, depression, and anxiety. They did much to render it possible to treat people on an outpatient basis who would formerly have been handled as inpatients, and they made more feasible the increased use of general instead of mental hospitals.

During the same period, there were extremely active programs aimed at public education and raising money through voluntary contributions. Promoted mainly by mental health associations, these programs were exceedingly successful in utilizing the media to bring mental health as a human problem to the attention of very large numbers of people.

Despite such achievements, major doubts and disillusionment about the mental health movement began to appear after the mid-sixties. By 1975, only 591 community mental health centers had been created in the United States, in contrast to the projected 2,000. Of these, only 443 were actually in operation.[5] The Nixon administration made efforts to abandon the mental health program, and President Ford originally vetoed legislation to amend the Community Mental Health Centers Act in 1974.[6]

Although Canada never had a national mental health centers program, it did have a mental health movement that took various shapes in different provinces. Some of the programs, as in Nova Scotia and Saskatchewan, were distinguished for boldness of conception, common sense, and some remarkable successes. But in Canada, too, countertrends arose.

Many of the doubts on both sides of the border stemmed from a widening of cracks lying within the movement from the start, as outlined in Chapter 3. These included increasing disharmony between psychiatrists and the other mental health workers over who should do what along with disagreements in all groups about the meaning of *mental health* and the best means for achieving whatever it was. Other doubts had to do with feasibility and costs, as the realization that there were large numbers of people in the population with various kinds of mental illnesses spread.[7] These doubts particularly affected programs for prevention and for fostering "positive mental health." The goal of providing services for everyone with a psychological or social need began to seem more and more like trying to drink the ocean.

The programs aimed at public education and the propaganda intended to encourage voluntary contributions almost certainly helped create disillusionment by raising expectations too high. Some of the statements were certainly extreme and appear to have been born of a willingness to say anything at a given moment that would generate support for the cause. They also exhibited a type of nonlogical lump thinking studded with slogans and appeals to the emotions that masked the stubborn issues summarized in Chapter 2. The issues were actually far more complex and difficult than the public and the legislators were led to believe.

The new medications, for example, successful as they were, brought new problems and an attending constellation of complex requirements. This was partly because many patients had to be kept on maintenance doses, much as diabetics must be kept on insulin, and also because some of the drugs could do serious damage unless dietary restrictions were observed and combinations with other drugs avoided. Neurological disabilities in facial muscles and limb control (tardive dyskinesia), blindness (retinitis pigmentosa), hypertensive crisis, and sudden death were some of the risks. These argued not only for knowledge, skill, and careful monitoring by the staffs of mental health centers, but also for meticulous communication among all physicians engaged in the care of any given patient in order to avoid overdosage or incompatible combinations of medications and in order to pick up, at the earliest possible moment, signs of damaging side effects.

The fact that drugs could be, and sometimes were, used to the detriment of patients led to the formation of groups hostile to their use in any way. The issue became ideological and emotional; the philosophical, religious, and cultist underpinnings of the debate called to mind the campaigns that had once raged against anesthetics and vaccinations.

Those who questioned the efficacy of treating mental illnesses were further encouraged by the fact that numerous epidemiological studies showed the highest prevalence rates to be in the economically poorest segments of the population. Under such circumstances, it was questioned whether care could amount to anything more than making individuals feel better temporarily before sending them back to the environments that had caused their disorders in the first place. To some people, it seemed that the proper answer was not clinical treatment but reform of the environment, that is, of society itself.

Nondrug therapies also burgeoned during the period under review and took shape as competing factions, helping to fragment the mental health movement and to increase doubts about it in the minds of policymakers. According to Stone:

The Fifties saw a schism between the dogmatically psychoanalytic and the dogmatically organic. During the Sixties, however, psychiatry moved from these polarities and became a conglomerate. Psychoanalysis lost much of its prestige and authority, and diverse schools of psychotherapy emerged – transactionalists, existentialists, gestaltists, and so forth. The behavior therapists, the sex therapists, the family therapists, and the group therapists all staked new claims. The behaviorist analysis of mental illness and its treatment became particularly powerful and influential.[8]

With the increasing numbers of different kinds of therapies, tensions accelerated in the changing relationships among the professions involved in the mental health movement. These were augmented by the philosophy of consumer participation. There was also more participation by sociologists and social psychologists, especially in the realm of theory. In the mental hygiene movement, as we have seen, it had been customary for a psychiatrist to be in charge of any unit that offered treatment to mentally ill persons. In the mental health movement, however, alternate and more egalitarian forms emerged in which a unit director could be a psychologist, a social worker, or a nurse or in which there might be no real director at all but, instead, some pattern of self-government. In the course of these changes, much struggling took place among the professions, with each endeavoring to establish a stronger identity, to achieve greater recognition, and to win a realm for independent action. The result was the further dilution of consensus regarding goals and activities for mental health centers and an increase in problems of defining and maintaining standards.

Amid all this turmoil, certain clinicians promoted the notion that mental illness is a myth, a product of socially shared but nevertheless false beliefs.[9] Similar views were also propounded by a number of social scientists.[10] It need hardly be said that the effect of these views was generally disorienting and widely disconcerting. When the Nova Scotia Council of Health published its report entitled *Health Care in Nova Scotia: A New Direction for the Seventies*, it stated that it had requested the views of all relevant psychiatric organizations and departments and had received, in addition, briefs from private practitioners. The upshot is described thus: "We have found this process frustrating. As a result of the inconsistency of the views expressed, basic contradiction and disagreements, we have no clear feeling of consensus on priorities and direction of this field."[11]

Concerned about the survival of community mental health in 1978, Borus drew attention to such issues as boundaries and priorities, caring for the chronically ill, relating to the rest of psychiatry and medicine, defining the community psychiatrist's role, and undertaking evaluation research.[12]

Writing from the perspective of 1980, Judd Marmur said that the "third revolution" in psychotherapy represents, for the most part, a radical departure from the scientific tradition.

It embraces a wide variety of approaches that reject the "mechanistic" view of man they attribute to both the psychoanalytic and the behavioral schools of thought. Under the broad umbrella of what has become known as the "human potential movement" these therapies focus on ways of achieving "peak" experiences, expanding consciousness, getting in touch with the "true self," releasing repressed emotions, experiencing what are presumed to be eternal verities, and "merging with the cosmos" by way of transcendental experiences.[13]

Such trends made it exceedingly difficult for the staff and Board of the Bristol Centre, the provincial government, and the Stirling County Study to foster orderliness and responsibility in patient care at the Centre and, even more, to maintain interest in scientific research. The goals and purposes of the mental health movement that had seemed clear in the fifties became murky in the seventies.

The medical profession

The medical profession during the period under consideration experienced changes that were no less significant to the goals of the Bristol Mental Health Centre than the trends just described in the mental health movement. These can be understood as an altering of relationships among three different categories of health-care delivery in which the medical profession is involved, each of which calls for a distinctive social structure and a different set of shared sentiments:

1   *Private services.* In these, the doctor places knowledge and skills at
     the disposal of all who can pay. The doctor acts as an independent
     private business run within a framework of professional ethics.

2   *Charitable services.* These arise because not all the people who want
     and need treatment can afford private services. Charitable services
     are, therefore, a humane supplement to private services and can be di-
     vided into four categories: free or low-cost aid given voluntarily by
     doctors in private practice; free or low-cost service given by medical
     schools and their affiliated hospitals in return for "teaching materi-
     als"; free or low-cost services given by religious or lay charities to un-
     derprivileged populations; and services given by government agencies,
     for example, mental hospitals and general health care for disadvan-
     taged groups such as Indians and Inuits.

3   *Public services.* In these, society through its government accepts the
     principle that every individual in the population has a right to health
     care. Thus, an ethic of rights replaces the ethic of charity, and the ori-
     entation of public service replaces that of private enterprise. This
     means that medical care is expected to reach not only those individu-
     als who realize they need help and know how to get it but also those
     who, through ignorance, discrimination, the nature of the disease, or
     other barriers, are failing to receive the attention they require.

Beginning at least as far back as the progressive era that followed the
conclusion of the nineteenth century, medical care in North America has
been moving unevenly from private services to public services. Encouraged by the Great Depression of the thirties, the trend gained force after
World War II. As everyone knows, each step of the way has been fraught
with controversy, ideological conflict, confrontations, and economic
problems.[14] By and large, the impetus for the shift has come from outside
the medical profession and has taken shape in government actions,
whereas resistance has come most strongly from within the profession,
particularly from the medical societies. This resistance is exemplified by
the Saskatchewan doctors' strike of 1962. Blishen, who was research director of the Royal Commission on Health Services and who made an
intensive and extensive study of physician views in Canada said, "professional control over the conditions of work is the most persistent concern
of the profession . . . closely followed by freedom of the physician and
the individual patient, and the quality of medical care."[15] The greatest
danger to these ideals was seen to be the government control that would
come with universal insurance and the intrusion of laymen into positions
of power in medical affairs. Blishen continues:

To accuse the medical profession of selfishness in attempting to protect its interests in the face of changes demanded by persons and groups outside the profession or to accuse it of ignorance of the effects of social change on the organization

and content of medical care is to over-simplify the nature of the difficulties facing the medical profession today . . . *All professions attempt to maintain control over their conditions of work as they interact with outsiders.*[16] [Emphasis added.]

The social structures and sentiments that develop in relation to private, charitable, and public services are often incompatible. Efforts to resolve conflict by compromise have meant that physicians find themselves participating in all three systems simultaneously and, hence, in contradictions and role confusions. For example, if as in Canada a general practitioner is paid on a fee-for-service basis, does that mean he is still, for all intents and purposes, in private practice? Or does he now have public health responsibilities? If so, what are they? As Woods has observed:

While governments, through such channels as former Minister of National Health and Welfare Marc Lalonde's "A New Perspective on the Health of Canadians," call for a new emphasis on preventive medicine, MD's probably best able to provide it – family physicians – are financially penalized for doing so. For example, a GP can perform a routine check-up on a patient in 10 or 15 minutes: if he spends another 20 minutes talking about smoking, exercise, diet and lifestyle influences on health and illness not a cent more is earned.[17]

McDermott has drawn attention to the fact that it may be impossible to offer readily available access to all persons in need simultaneously and also to take the necessary time with each individual patient required to ensure that technologically correct medical care is given together with whatever human support is indicated.[18]

Reactions within the medical profession to these role stresses and role confusions have been numerous and varied. Crises of leadership have occurred, together with the breakup of many formerly shared sentiments, often marked by lowering of professional morale. Strikes have already been mentioned, but an alternative reaction is for members of the profession to close ranks and withdraw from other subsystems of society such as government agencies and lay boards. It is a common observation that a group under stress will try to purify itself and strive for solidarity against perceived dangers. The process has a high potential for taking precedence over other considerations such as general civic good or the provision of quality care.

In such a climate of feeling, the position of the psychiatrist can be precarious. Often regarded as "not a real doctor," he can be asked to show his medical colors and stand firmly within the closed ranks, or he can be defined as an outsider who is busy about mental health and who consorts on equal terms with lay people and with social workers, psychologists, and other nonmedical and therefore suspect types of healers.

This turmoil in the medical profession and the trends within the mental health movement combined during the period of our case study to place many obstacles in the way of institutions such as the Bristol Centre whose goals depended on coordination among professions and cooperation with various nonprofessional organizations and agencies of government – town, county, provincial, and federal.

The sick society

The problems of the mental health movement and of the medical profession were rendered more disorderly and difficult to manage by an overwhelming popular surge of sentiments in the sixties condemning in sweeping terms the institutions and values of Western society.

The notion that society is evil and unjust is at least as old in European history as the notion of sin. That evil social processes can play a role in causing, precipitating, or perpetuating mental illnesses has been a seriously entertained idea for centuries and was highlighted during the era of moral treatment. It was also, as we have seen in Chapter 3, a component of the mental hygiene movement and was carried over into the mental health movement. From being a social and research issue of interest mainly to mental health workers and social scientists in the fifties, the theories about psychological damage being inflicted by social conditions became transmuted during the sixties into a popular ideology about which there were soon very strong feelings. As if experiencing a revelation, a great many people became convinced that it was society that was sick, not individuals. This conviction constituted a remarkable flowing together of political radicalism and psychiatric and social science theories. The consequent impact on policies, legislation, plans, and services for people with mental illnesses was profound.

The late sixties was a period of rage over the Vietnam war, during which many young Americans fled to Canada, of spreading drug use, of "sexual revolution," and of a youth movement and a counterculture in opposition to the way of life theretofore dominant in Canada, the United States, Europe, and much of the rest of the world where industrialization, technological development, and material wealth had been either the aspiration or the accomplishment.[19] The members of the counterculture decried such evils as the rich–poor dichotomy; pollution of the earth, the seas, and the air; the degradation of human values by a machine-dominated technology; wars around the world that never ended; the strangling grip of bureaucracy on individual freedom; the exploitative immorality of advertising and industrial management; the use of the "big lie" in politics;

and much else, but overall and finally, the hovering threat of nuclear destruction, which, as they saw it, was the outstanding contribution of science.

A variety of apparently reactive behaviors was associated with these views. One extreme sought disengagement from the web of worldly interactions and tried to make inner being and feeling all in all, with or without the use of drugs, music, transcendental meditation, and various cult memberships. Efforts to escape also took the form of intoxication through excitement by means of roving and sex, after the fashion of Jack Kerouac, and by committing crimes for thrill, like the Manson gang.[20]

Another extreme sought active engagement in attack upon the existing state of affairs. The long-range goal was said to be reform of society, but the immediate need was seen as the destruction of the "whole system" so that new freedom and a far, far better way of life could emerge. It was in the service of this goal that protests, strikes, building occupations, and property destruction took place all over North America. Damage to the amount of $2½ million was done to the computer equipment in the Sir George Williams Institute in Montreal, and a research laboratory in Wisconsin was blown up. It was the era of the Weathermen, symbolizing and expressing in dramatic action the widespread sentiments of individualism, of rights, and of hostility toward elite groups, toward virtually all forms of social control, and toward many of the traditional values that had hitherto been incorporated in conceptions of mental health.

A group representing a significant development in Canada, the Company of Young Canadians, went through one of its important early phases at a place not very far from the Bristol Mental Health Centre. This was its first training session, conducted in June of 1966 at Crystal Cliffs near Antigonish, Nova Scotia. The Company of Young Canadians, created by the federal government in the mid-sixties, embodied many of the ideas of the Peace Corps and Vista in the United States. It went further, however, in a policy of giving young people a free hand to set their own objectives and to bring about social change even if it meant disrupting "the establishment." The first ten days of the training session were occupied with a "human relations laboratory" run by a psychiatrist from one of the province's mental health centers.

The aims of the group were stated to be "seeking a society in which people are in charge of their own destinies. Second, we seek a society in which diversity and variety are the basis of human life."[21] Summing up the document that describes the aims and principles of the group, Hamilton said, "In the rhetoric of the left, it slams at the liberals (do-gooders) and at the agencies (the bandage boys). It sets up the framework for participatory democracy and self-determination."[22]

The columnist and former New Democratic Party member, Douglas Fisher, observed:

A further belief of the volunteer is that the sickness of society is more manifest in the exploiters than in the exploited. Who are the exploiters? The middle class, the politicians, the men and women who staff the schools and government departments – all bureaucrats . . .

When I asked one young lady, who will be working with Indians and Eskimos, if she had talked with any experts in the field, she wrinkled her nose and said: "Never, they've been oppressing the Indians and the Eskimos for a century. They'll be my enemy."[23]

From such a beginning, the Company went on to a career of some quiet successes and many stormy episodes, with virtually constant internal turmoil. In the fall of 1969, officials in the city of Montreal appealed to the Prime Minister to institute a royal commission to investigate the activities of the Company. The reasons they gave included the following: some Company members had been convicted of participating in terrorist activities, had been helping to organize protest marches and class boycotts by college and university students, and had in their offices piles of communist propaganda and revolutionary instructions on how to make Molotov cocktails, bombs, and other weapons.

The Company of Young Canadians leaves scars on people. It was, and probably still is, an organization driven by emotion, with personality pitted against personality. It was an organization where battles to the death were an everyday occurrence, where compromise showed weakness – a view typical of civil service.

I suffered and bled with CYC for more than two years. I too was changed by the time I left. Instead of being calm and mild, I found myself edgy, attuned to crisis situations, and used to fighting – continuous fighting."[24]

The Company of Young Canadians illustrates the widespread sentiments of the time that emphasized instant solutions to human problems by adversary and advocacy procedures and by demand and confrontation. To a large extent, the mood was both ahistorical and opposed to fact gathering and to applying scientific methods to human affairs. There was little inclination for a balanced analysis of just what aspects of society might be "sick" and in what ways it might also be considered "healthy." One heard much about "this repressive society of ours" as the embodiment of evil but little about how it actually compared in the repressive dimension with its behavior in former times or with other societies in the contemporary world. Nor was there assessment in comparative terms of the degree to which permissiveness might be, in fact, one of its unusual, and possibly harmful, features.

An outside observer might have concluded that the middle class in

North America was caught up in an orgy of self-hate, such as is sometimes seen in religious conversion, and was impelled by some kind of emotional necessity to confess a great burden of sins, both real and unreal. The emotional intensity, the simplistic ideology, and the high educational level and caliber of some of the people involved was more than a little reminiscent of the spiritualism movement a hundred years before. The inequalities and injustices of society were, of course, real, horrifying, and in need of correction, just as they have been for centuries if not forever.

The sixties can be credited with the development of an unusually keen degree of social awareness, but the solutions adopted were often nonrational and magical. The feeling climate of the time favored those emotional reactions that I described in Chapter 2 as the second of the four major barriers to progress in dealing with mental illnesses. It also, of necessity, favored barrier three – the nonuse of science – in marked contrast to the hopes of the early fifties, which had focused on the social sciences.

The repercussions of the sentiments of the sixties for the medical profession were numerous. Medicine was criticized for its detachment from human issues, for "elitism," and for running its services for the benefit of doctors and nurses rather than patients. Psychiatry, in particular, came under attack for misapplying "the medical model" to what were essentially "human problems" that demanded change in social conditions. In the opinion of some people, the nature of mental illness called on the psychiatrist to separate from medicine and espouse revolution.

A number of psychiatrists did just this, turning from the research and development goals of social psychiatry to political action. They sought the mitigation of stressful conditions through attacks on race and sex prejudices, on poverty, on restrictions of individual freedom, and in general on the management of human affairs by the "establishment."

Within the American Psychiatric Association, individuals and groups participated in various kinds of demonstrations at the annual meetings, often disrupting scientific papers. So disturbed were matters that this professional society found it necessary on occasion to have police check the credentials of everybody seeking admission to its meetings. In Montreal, at a psychiatric dinner, Dr. Richard Kunner sprayed creamwhip over Dr. Heinz Lehmann, declaring that practicing psychiatry in the society of today is about as corrupt as being a psychiatrist in a concentration camp.[25]

Extremists looked on psychiatric treatment as "brainwashing," as conditioning deviants to the requirements of a "repressive society." This seemed to be an echo of the well-known Communist view that religion is the opiate of the masses. It was said that the real trouble was that a sick society was either forcing people into so-called abnormal behavior or, by focusing on individualistic behaviors (to which a person had an inalienable right) was stereotyping and labeling these as mental illness and then proceeding to cast the person in the "sick role." Freedom became the watchword, freedom from discrimination and freedom from labels, especially psychiatric labels. As Stone put it:

The scene was Miami Beach, 1969. The American Psychiatric Association had gathered for its annual meeting. Overhead a small plane droned back and forth. Behind it a sign fluttered. Its legend: "Psychiatry Kills." That message reflects fear of a therapeutic state, a clockwork-orange vision of citizens drugged and bugged by the psychiatric establishment. It unites the far left and the far right in a shared nightmare of political dissenters transmogrified into madmen by conspiratorial psychiatrists.[26]

Stone goes on to say that the viewpoint represented by the slogan "Psychiatry Kills" found immediate allies among lawyers concerned about civil liberties.

The notion that a person was mentally ill became a nasty and derogatory approach to be rejected by courts, which instead were to apply legal standards and legal safeguards.

An important legal precedent was set when a Michigan court found, among other things, that psychosurgery might by interfering with the brain, interfere with mentation and thus interfere with the First Amendment. Given that precedent and the legal analysis on which it was based, civil libertarians moved to extend that reasoning and to control electro-shock treatment, behavior therapy and tranquilizers. Many of the most significant developments in the treatment of the seriously mentally ill were to be hedged in by complicated legal restraints. The sentiment that psychiatric treatment is either brain damaging or brainwashing was implicit in all of these legal developments.

The legend "Psychiatry Kills" was replaced by the epitaph "Psychiatry is Dead." This became a rallying cry for many different social factions – those who have always despised psychiatry (among them many physicians who are unnerved by the Freudian view of the inherent fallibility of human nature); members of competing mental professions who have always chafed at the special status of psychiatrists; and government bureaucrats who, whether in the name of "Psychiatry Kills" or "Psychiatry is Dead," hoped to save dollars by doing away with mental health care.[27]

Parallel with these trends was the turbulence on the university and college campuses of North America, soon followed by troubles in the secondary schools, including the schools of Stirling County. As reported by Herbers,[28] from the beginning of November 1968 to the end of February 1969, there were 239 serious episodes of "strikes, sit-ins, demonstrations, riots or other violence" in high schools. Blackmer quoted a national survey of secondary school principals in the United States as reporting student protests in 67 percent of American city and suburban schools.[29] A Canadian review and analysis of such problems found it "obvious" that the trend was very similar in Canada, although no figures were given.[30]

The topical foci of these troubles were such matters as lack of student influence in shaping school rules and policies, poor communication between students and faculty (including administrations), dress and hair codes, and lack of relevance of what was taught to the real world. The students were described as feeling themselves to be a "new breed" and to be "tense, frustrated and on edge."[31]

Lipset emphasized a "backlash opposition to systematic and quantitative social science, to large scale social research, to the very conception of the utility of efforts at objective scholarship . . . and the concomitant belief in gradualism, expertise, and planning."[32] These comments refer to college and university campuses, but they doubtless apply to the high schools as well.

In terms of emotional quality, anger, demand, and blaming are, of course, apparent. Hobart gave particular emphasis to "hatred," and Blackmer mentioned boredom because of rigid daily schedules.[33]

The leadership and integration of the high school protests is seen by some authors as indigenous and reactive to intolerable situations,[34] whereas others took more note of outside influences. Thus, Hobart thought that "the leaders may – at times – be young, popular, vigorous teachers, who have strong leanings toward activism from their own university days. Or they may be university students, seeking to attract broader support for a particular demonstration, or to promote increased activism at high schools."[35]

Both psychiatry and the social sciences contributed to the stock of beliefs employed by the social activists. These included the ideas that repression of anger is destructive to personality, that all cultural values are relative and so a matter of individual choice, that society creates mental illness by forcing people into sick roles and labeling them, and that almost everybody has within him or her potential for self-realization that is destroyed by conformity to the norms and demands of "our society." Most of these beliefs had their origins in work that was genuinely scientific. They were theories or parts of theories developed as guides to empirical investigations that would, by degrees, support, modify, develop, or reject them.

Psychological, social, and cultural theories often engage the public's interest, and there are both social scientists and media writers who enjoy translating them into terms the public comprehends. In this process (which usually involves reification, dramatization, and omission of qualifications), theories lose their tentative characters and appear as "scientific findings," soon translated into ideologies and articles of political faith. In this form and usage, they are, of course, no longer scientific, even though a scientific aura may be retained and play a part in their credibility. The have lost their function as way stations on the road to accumulating more and more useful knowledge and have become, instead, ammunition in ideological wars.

Turbulence in Bristol: the school issue

The description given up to this point of what was occurring in society at large across North America amounts to a set of abstractions that represents multiple, local realities. Although these realities must have varied considerably from place to place, it may be doubted whether any village, town, or city was entirely unaffected.

In order to give some of the facts and flavor of one such cluster of local realities, I shall describe an instance of turbulence occurring in the Bristol schools. Because the Mental Health Centre was involved, some of my colleagues and I observed and recorded as many as possible of the events and interviewed a number of the participants. Like much of the rest of the case study, the data gathered contain material focused on persons and personalities as well as information derived from confidential sources. In order to report and yet remain within the bounds of ethical considerations, I have in the synopsis that follows utilized material that is already in the public domain, mostly in newspapers. The selection, however, has been conducted in such a way as to make the whole remain in line with the private sources of information and thus give, as far as possible, an accurate – even if only partial – account of what happened.

On November 13, 1969, a young, recently hired teacher in the Bristol school system, a newcomer to the area, wrote a letter to a local paper. He called for regular, open school board meetings that would welcome the attendance of teachers and parents, active Home and School Associations (the Canadian equivalent of PTA) at every school, representatives of teachers' unions on school boards, and other such reforms.

In reviewing events a year later, another newspaper, the *Mysterious East* (December 1970), which had a revolutionary philosophy, observed that the teacher's prior involvement in a "bus strike dispute did not serve to endear him to the educational establishment." It added, "It seems clear, in fact, that at this point of his career he was not a very good teacher. It is possible that some of his unhappiness with the system was due to this. But it is also clear that there are many worse teachers."

On November 21, 1969, the teacher received a registered letter from the superintendent of schools, which said, in part:

I have been instructed by the Bristol Regional School Board to advise you that the Board by unanimous resolution decided to terminate your contract, to become effective November 30, 1969. The reason for this action by the Board is unsatisfactory performance of your probationary contract.

The recipient of the letter exercised his right to appeal and the school board extended his salary pending the outcome of the hearing. Division of opinion as to whether the teacher or the school administration was in the right ran through the town and municipal councils, several other school boards, the teacher's union, the students, the Mental Health Association, and the Mental Health Centre Board, as well as the population at large. The staff of the Mental Health Centre, on the other hand, was not divided, but sided strongly with the teacher.

What is remarkable is not the fact that a difference of opinion arose but rather the degree to which it soon became charged with strong, angry emotions. Very early, the controversy took on the coloring of a struggle between those who favored the "establishment" and those who favored youth and the kind of revolutionary sentiments expressed by the Company of Young Canadians.

The provincial government set up a commission composed of three lawyers from outside the Bristol area to review the teacher's appeal. On January 20, 1970, this body reached a decision in his favor and ordered his reinstatement. The three top members of the school administration – the superintendent of schools, the supervisor of schools, and the high school principal – thereupon resigned. Emotional tension heightened in the town and its surrounding area. Some people felt they had won an important victory and that with this advantage they should move quickly to bring about further changes they desired. Others felt that a serious injustice had been done to the school administrators and that steps must be taken to prevent a catastrophe in the educational system.

An editorial appeared on January 28 in a local paper, the main part of which said:

The recent controversy in the Bristol school system . . . and discussions of rallying to the support of one side or another, has not been good publicity for the fine town of Bristol.

We are not taking sides in the matter, and will not do so, but will continue to see that the welfare of the students and our children is given top priority.

Where we do express concern is over the welfare of students and children. With the rallying of one side against another, which is possible, by parents or teachers, the only ones to suffer seriously will be the students.

About this time, the reinstated teacher wrote the following letter to the school board:

Dear Sirs:

I understand from the *Chronicle-Herald* [a Halifax newspaper] that the Superintendent of the Bristol Regional School System has resigned, effective July, 1970.

Obviously the office is open and applications for appointment to the position will be accepted by you and considered on the merits and qualifications of the candidates for appointment to this position . . .

I now submit with all sincerity my application for appointment to the Office of Superintendent of Schools in the Bristol Regional School System.

I am not the best qualified person. He is a man about my age between 30 and 40 years old, now employed in Ontario, who has a M.E. or M.A. (educ.) and experience as a principal. I do not know his name, residence, color, or where he is now employed. I should prefer that he be appointed instead of me.

Nevertheless, at this time we do not know who he is and until then, I request that you carefully consider my application.

Respectfully submitted,

Copies of this letter were sent to the local papers, the chairperson of the school board, the Bristol Municipal School Board, and the president of the teachers' union local. Many individuals thought the letter odd, given the circumstances, and expressive of a very curious kind of thinking.

Also about this time, a ten-member "citizens' committee" formed itself at a meeting in a black village situated several miles outside the town of Bristol. The following excerpts are taken from the January 28 issue of a local paper.

Approximately 60 people were in attendance at the meeting, which was called to discuss common problems faced by parents of students in the Bristol and area school system.

It should be noted here that the alleged discrimination was not one of a racial nature, but of a general discriminatory basis.

The attendance of the meeting was approximately half Negro; the remaining half, whites from various areas contained in the Bristol school system.

At the meeting, Mrs. X said she went to talk to the administrative staff concerning a child of hers in the school. Mrs. X stated that she met with them for four hours and about all they could say was "We feel this, and we feel that." Mrs. X said she told the administrative staff she couldn't care how they felt, all she was concerned about was her child.

Mrs. X stated in summarizing her statement, "They felt all afternoon and I didn't feel a thing."

Shortly after the formation of the citizens' committee, its chairperson reported at a meeting that he and other members had received threatening phone calls. He denied rumors, which he said were circulating, that the committee was planning to bring in Black Panthers. Following this, numbers of people on both sides of the school issue reported threatening calls, and some were so bothered that they secured unlisted telephone numbers.

An indication of the emotional intensity involved at this point is the fact that a bridge tournament to raise money for the Curling Club was canceled because the sponsors thought there would be too many people who would refuse to play together. The condition of the town began to resemble Hamilton's description of the Company of Young Canadians as "driven by emotion, with personality pitted against personality . . . where compromise showed weakness."

During the early part of February 1970, an agreement was reached between the reinstated teacher and the school board whereby he formally resigned and moved away from the area but continued to receive his salary until the end of the school year.

A few days later, a local paper reported a petition that asked the three school administrators who had resigned to reconsider their decisions. At a heavily attended meeting of the teachers' union local, the union executives, who had been favorable to the teacher's case, were forced out of office by the members and replaced with a new group. After having thus repudiated its former leaders, the local then voted to support the three administrators.

On the 28th of February, some 600 people gathered to ask once more that the three administrators reconsider. Two of them did so, but the superintendent of schools changed his position only from resignation to retirement in the coming summer.

The mayor of Bristol appealed to the public, saying, "I beg you to let the situation calm down."

On this same day, the *Chronicle-Herald* reported that the teachers were greatly concerned about the education of the students and indicated their willingness to cooperate with the administration and the school boards in resolving any conflicts that might remain. The newspaper also reported the teachers as saying that they would not participate in community pressure groups or committees "pro or con."

Yet, on Tuesday, March 3, the same paper featured an article under the banner headline "Education Crisis Divides People of Bristol." It said that the town was divided into two camps, neither side "looking for a common ground that might end the quarrelling and distrust." The superintendent was described as the "driving force in the system since 1961." The article continued:

When schools became overcrowded and outdated, it was he who pushed best and hardest for money to build additions and new schools. When high school education was regionalized, it was he who pushed for construction of Bristol Regional High School.

When he was not looking after school business, he took care of problems of the town's hospital, and is the hospital board chairman. He also found time to push through the construction of the new 96-bed hospital, the latest in a series and not the first that bore his mark.

His drive has made him the central and dominant character in the town's two most important industries: education and healing.

The article puzzled over the reasons why the superintendent's resignation had aroused so much controversy and said that the chairperson of the school board "candidly admitted last weekend that he doesn't know."

His own problem is the high school teaching staff, among whom the issue caused a rift a mile wide. He is not sure what the problems are there either, except that young teachers want changes.

The Chairperson said further that he wants both sides to work out their differences because the students are suffering. Two of the three academic senior grades had below normal results in recent midterm examinations.

The leader of the citizens' committee is quoted as saying "the superintendent has wielded too much power and is still doing so . . . his actions are dictatorial." The superintendent must go, he said, and so must the other two administrators because "they have been too close to the Superintendent and have become tainted." The article ended by saying, "there appeared little hope of compromise, little chance of ending the bitterness."

People who thought progress was being made toward resolution were profoundly upset by the article. They felt that it overemphasized extremist views, encouraged the hardening of positions, discouraged negotiation, and gave to "agitators" the notice they were ardently seeking. Many believed that the town would be much better able to handle its affairs if it could avoid the glare of metropolitan publicity that was seen as the work of outsiders intent on profiting from the local troubles.

About mid-March, the school board announced that two teachers who had been in active opposition to the administration would not have their contracts renewed in the coming year. One of these had been a member of the deposed executive board of the teachers' union local. On March 17 and 18, students at the school staged a sit-down and then a protest march in favor of retaining the two teachers. Not all students participated; some 600 out of about 900 carried on as usual, and, according to a local paper, numbers of those who did participate were not sure why they were marching. The president of the student council was not himself a participant, and he told the paper that the student council was divided in its opinion about the protest.

The protesters maintained that the demonstration was "100 percent" a student affair. Some people noted, however, that refreshments had been prepared in advance by adults at a place convenient for the marchers to rest, and the citizens' committee was accused of having encouraged, if not having instigated, the protest.

During the two protest days, a group of the students attempted to take over the local radio station, but eventually desisted when the station personnel managed to lock themselves in and the students out. The station director said later that he finally had to go off the air because of "kids pounding on the windows, shaking the door, and even climbing on the roof."

An incident occurred during the march that reflected both the high pitch of excitement and the muddled ideology of the crisis. A Jewish merchant standing in front of his store and watching the parade go by was suddenly the target of anti-Semitic abuse from a black boy.

On March 24, the annual school dance was interrupted and disbanded due to a telephone warning that a bomb had been planted – the first of a long series of telephoned scares that greatly disturbed the schools.

About the middle of March, a three-man survey team appointed by the minister of education for Nova Scotia held thirty-four individual interviews in the course of a two-week period. The report was released on the first of April and was carried in a local paper the next day under the headline "Rivalries in Community Cloud Real School Issues, Solution Must Come from Community."

The report described the situation as complex and emotional and added that "the emotional atmosphere in which it developed gave it greater proportions than it should ever have assumed." The paper reported the following:

Further commenting on specific complaints, it was revealed by the report that there is every indication that over the years a very strong school system has been established under the leadership of the superintendent. He had made a tremendous contribution to the development of education in the area and the value of his service should be given public recognition, the report stated.

In respect to the complaints relating to the difficulty in obtaining answers from the administration, the team found that they did occur, but not to the extent that has been indicated.

The administration, at all times, were conscious of the taxpayers' dollars and instituted economies whenever and wherever they could, the report revealed.

It appeared to the team that generally, all who came before the survey team were motivated by a sincere desire to work for the welfare of the children and their concerns were legitimate. A few, however, the report said, appeared to be prompted by personal interests which gave no consideration to the well-being of the community. Quoting from the report: "At times it appeared as if the basic needs of the students were often ignored in the conflicting points of view expressed by adults, and what is still more serious, one suspected that the students themselves were being used and manipulated to add strength to some individuals' presentation to the survey team."

A high degree of rigidity has characterized the functioning of the school administration, a situation which has deteriorated during the past few years. This was found to be the root of the current school problems, the survey said. The taxpayer consistently had been refused quick and easy access to information which is his right to have; many parents had been unable to communicate with the teachers and administration in a normal, relaxed way; and several teachers likewise had experienced frustration in communicating with the administration, were some of the complaints by those interviewed.

The financial operations of the administration had been most satisfactory; however, financial considerations while an important factor, should only be a major concern after all educational implications have been studied, the survey indicated.

The Bristol school administration, under the direction of the Superintendent, in the view of the survey, assumed far too much responsibility for detail in respect to the operation and administration of the school system, and because they did assume and take over practically all of the detail, the work load became such that they could not easily keep the school boards fully informed of the decisions and actions.

Presently in the Bristol school system, there seems to be no clear definition of the respective duties of Superintendent, Supervisor, and to some extent, Principal of the high school. The survey report recommended that these be spelled out in order to avoid any duplication of function.

This effort at balanced judgment and fair play was followed by one of a different kind from the Canadian Broadcasting Corporation television show "Weekend" that was transmitted coast to coast. Charlotte Gobeil presented the school issue as a dramatic struggle of the underdog against the establishment. Much more time was given to those who attacked the school and other leadership than to those who explained alternative points of view. The effect was to help keep things boiling in the area, generating glee and also outrage over injustice and falsehood.

During April and May, the turmoil began to lessen, which was probably related to the actual or imminent departure of several persons who had been involved in the protest movement. The chairperson of the citizens' committee moved to another province, and, as we have seen, two of the activist teachers had been refused new contracts by the school board and so had signed with schools in other parts of Nova Scotia. The teacher whose grievance had precipitated the crisis had already left.

The quiet, however, was by no means complete. There were still those who thought that an important struggle to change the schools was being lost. Among these were staff members of the Mental Health Centre, and they published letters in the papers aimed at arousing the public and keeping the school issue alive. In contrast to these were others who wanted to see the fight continued for the sake of the fun and excitement it provided. As a consequence, many persons were on tenterhooks lest trouble break out again.

On the 23rd of April, at a meeting that filled the school auditorium to capacity, a Home and School Association was formed and a physician was elected president. The general spirit of the meeting was optimistic, and there were hopes for the reestablishment of good feelings. No members of the Mental Health Centre staff were present.

At the high school graduating exercise in June, the school board chairman made a presentation to the retiring superintendent, who was given a standing ovation by the graduates and audience. On August 23, a dinner attended by more than 300 people was held for the retiring superintendent as a means of recognizing and showing appreciation for "all he had done" for the people of the region, and especially for the generations of children who had passed through the school system. A number of individuals who had left the area returned in order to participate.

Alongside this account it is appropriate to lay a backward-looking comment by the teacher whose firing precipitated the crisis. As quoted in the *Mysterious East* in December 1970, he said that the school "was run like some of the prisons I've visited, humiliating students continuously, shaming them as much as possible, disallowing any creative activity or free discussion. In some respects it was much like a mental institution."

In an interview reported in the *Ottawa Citizen* on August 5, 1972, Charlotte Gobeil said she had been wrong in the view of the situation she had presented in the "Weekend" broadcast. She recalled this experience in order to illustrate her point in the interview that "not all advocacy of the oppressed turns out." According to the report, "She made a special trip to Bristol to interview a young American teacher charging the school principal and town people with persecution leading to dismissal. Too late came the realization that he had misrepresented the facts to suit himself."

As a step toward understanding some of the societal factors at work in the turbulence over the school issue, those of us who were engaged in the case study identified all the individuals on both sides who appeared to be exerting major influences. Our criteria for major influence were two: repeated public statements that were carried by press and radio; and/or occupying formal positions of leadership in local organizations. The number of "influentials" evident on this basis turned out to be twenty-four, equally divided between the two sides. Each of these influentials was then further identified in terms of age, sex, occupation, education, and years in Bristol or its vicinity. Although the exact age and educational level were not ascertained in every case, all the influentials were at least seen by one of us, and most relevant aspects of past history were obtained. We think, therefore, that in instances where estimates of age and level of education are used they cannot have been far off the mark and are not likely to affect our general conclusions.

The mean age of the twelve establishment influentials was 48, with a range from 36 to 65, whereas the mean age for the twelve opposition influentials was 42, with a range from 23 to 50. On the whole, therefore, the opposition was younger than the establishment, but not a great deal younger. Only four were 40 or under.

There was only one woman among the establishment influentials, whereas six of the twelve opposition influentials were women.

In order to compare the two groups in terms of socioeconomic class, we employed the Hollingshead Two Factor Index. The mean score for the establishment was 15.5, which places the group as a whole in Class I; the range was from Class I to Class III. The mean score for the opposition was 31, which places that group as a whole in Class III. The distribution for the opposition was as follows:

Class I	3 members
Class II	4 members
Class III	3 members
Class IV	0 members
Class V	2 members

It is apparent from this that, at least among the influentials, the school issue was a battle not between haves and have-nots but rather between two groups of haves, one of which was, on the average, composed of somewhat older and higher status haves than the other.

Analysis of place of birth reveals that neither group consisted mainly of natives of Bristol or its vicinity. On the establishment side, ten out of twelve were nonnatives, whereas in the opposition the figures were eleven out of twelve. On the other hand, the establishment and the opposition differed markedly in the amount of time members had lived in Bristol. The establishment influentials had a mean of 24 years of residence, with a range from 5 to 65 years, whereas the opposition had a mean of 12 years, with a range from less than 1 to 50 years. This comparison is, of course, affected by the age differences. If, however, one compares percentage of life in Bristol, the same kind of contrast between the two groups emerges. The establishment influentials had a mean of 50 percent, with a range from 13 to 100 percent, whereas the opposition had a mean of 28 percent, with a range from 3 to 100 percent.

It is apparent, therefore, that, insofar as the influentials can be used as indicators, the school issue was mainly a battle between new newcomers and old newcomers. It was not a revolt that sprang from the grass-roots natives of the area, either old or young, but was rather something precipitated by outsiders. Added evidence for this is the fact that five of the twelve opposition influentials had been in Bristol less than 2 years and, further, that these all left before another year had elapsed. Interestingly, the prime target of the opposition's attack, the superintendent, was a native.

One can therefore interpret the school issue as having been precipitated by an invasion – in one respect, an invasion by the sentiments characteristic of urban and suburban society in the late sixties, and in another respect, an invasion by actual individuals. The activists attracted support from other dissatisfied people in Bristol, many of them also newcomers. The motivations were complex, ranging from a genuine desire to bring about improvements to various forms of self-aggrandizement. A number of individuals, for example, found that by joining the opposition they became influentials for the first time in their lives. Of the twelve opposition influentials, ten had never had a position of influence in Bristol prior to this participation. Among the establishment influentials, only one could be described in these terms.

Our information also suggests that economic considerations played a role. Shaking up the school administration could be viewed as a way to create jobs at the top (see the fired teacher's letter applying for the position of superintendent), to open up possibilities for contractors and suppliers who had been excluded by the former school administration, and to reduce or prevent increases in property taxes by curtailing the planned further development of the educational system.

Finally, let us note that the Stirling County Study's analysis of the population in the study area during the early and mid-fifties had pointed to the presence of people with extreme "weakness of community attachment." These occurred both as social isolates and as small pockets of socioculturally disintegrated neighborhoods. In Bristol, the rate was estimated from a sampling survey as about 20 percent of the adults. Hughes et al. expressed the view that such people were dangerous both to themselves and others. They were said to be dangerous to themselves because of their apathy, or "anomie," and their inability to deal adequately with their social environment. The authors further said:

They are also dangerous to the larger society [because the area] might easily have its social system clogged by a rising tide of anomie and paralyzing disparagement, if present sociocultural trends continue.

Although these people are now almost leaderless and have very poor dispositions toward followership, it seems evident that . . . they could participate in violence more easily than they could in the tedious business of constructiveness.[36]

As has often been observed, young people from about fifteen to twenty years of age constitute a segment of the population that by and large has minimal attachment to the traditions and shared sentiments of their elders. Although they usually have very strong attachment to networks made up of their own age mates, they often have little commitment to the norms of the larger society. In this detachment, they resemble the socially disintegrated or isolated adults. In the sixties, as a result of the "baby boom" associated with World War II, they made up an unusually large proportion of the population.

The school issue, therefore, can be seen as in part an outbreak of fire ignited by outside influences among these accumulated inflammable human materials, a fire that was only contained after much suffering and serious difficulty and that threatened for a long time to break out again.

Crises in social systems

Outside influences were, of course, not the whole story in the turbulence generated by the school issue in Bristol. What they did was to make a tear in the town's social structure and in its network of shared sentiments. This led to a dissolution of many constraints and permitted a rowdy flow of preexisting emotions. Thus, although the tear occurred partly as a result of the strength of the invasion, it was also partly due to weaknesses in the town's shared sentiments and social organization, weaknesses that are characteristic of many if not all towns today and that will be discussed in Chapter 8. The confluence of outside influences and internal weaknesses resulted in a profound and extensive disequilibrium that was so disturbing to societal functioning that for a time it took on the proportions of a crisis.

Recurrent episodes of large and small crises are endemic in human societies, as can be well seen, for example, in the histories of the New England towns so often evoked as model communities. They had repeated social explosions, the most notorious of which resulted in the witchcraft trials at Salem.[37]

William Kornhauser has said that "you cannot understand what happens in a community in times of crisis by understanding what happens under routine conditions."[38] Basing his analysis on disputes that arose over fluoridation in community water supplies during the fifties, he also says that "those elements in a community that do *not* have power, win controversies." He explains this paradox by saying that, by and large, establishments do not fight vigorously in dealing with crises. In his experience, they

did not do so . . . because they did not want to alienate large numbers of people. You cannot fight very hard if you are a dentist, for example, because you lose those patients who are against fluoridation. You cannot fight very hard if you are a public official because you lose votes. The opponents of fluoridation, on the other hand, are generally those *without* commitments or responsibilities in the community and are therefore capable of putting on a much stronger fight. They are not exposed to the usual restraints on responsible people who have economic and political interests in the community . . .

The second observation I wish to call to your attention is that the anti-fluoridation group – and again this is very typical – treated fluoridation as a *conspiracy* . . . This belief in conspiracy is crucial; you will find it again and again in community controversies. The idea presented is that the "little people" are fighting against certain mysterious forces that can create havoc and destruction among us.

The third observation is this: the people who supported the anti-fluoridation group – this is based on a survey of voters before the election – were, on the average, those of less education, lower occupational status, and lower incomes.

The central factor is the strength or weakness of community attachment . . . Usually the lack of attachment to community groups leads to apathy, but under critical conditions it may lead to extremist responses.

Furthermore, people who do not participate in any way in the community are much less likely to understand what is going on, and this lack has particularly serious consequences. For when a crisis does appear and these people become involved in community controversy, their actions and opinions are not tempered by an understanding of the true nature of the situation. Thus you get highly irrational and extremist interpretations of events, such as the belief in a conspiracy.[39]

Slogans that make charges of conspiracy are effective in mobilizing support inasmuch as they rally people with grudges and grievances of all kinds. At the same time, they stifle opposition because those in positions of responsibility are anxious to show they are really not engaged in conspiracy, and, hence, they tend to remain silent and to refrain from posing barriers.

Coleman has been impressed by how much one crisis is like another: "The most striking fact about the development and growth of community controversies is the similarity they exhibit despite diverse underlying sources and different kinds of precipitating incidents."[40] The previously silent become highly vocal, and apathy vanishes into intensely felt polarization. Furthermore, it is very characteristic that the issues "which provide the initial basis of response in a controversy undergo great transformations."

As partisan organizations are formed and a real nucleus develops around each of the opposing centers, new leaders tend to take over the dispute; often they are men who have not been community leaders in the past, men who face none of the constraints of maintaining a previous community position, and feel none of the cross-pressures felt by members of community organizations.

The new leaders are seldom moderates; the situation itself calls for extremists. And such men have not been conditioned, through experience in handling past community problems, to the prevailing norms concerning tactics of dispute.[41]

All in all, crises are a period of far-ranging risk because they foster sociocultural disintegration, and, as a consequence, both bad and good service programs may be destroyed indiscriminately.

The crisis in Bristol gradually subsided, but at the time our case study of the Centre ended in 1972, it was smoldering rather than extinct. Many people were still afraid it would break out again.

Concluding note

One of the most significant changes observable in society at large between the fifties and the seventies was in roles and role relationships. Numerous roles became less easy to define and their areas of rights and responsibilities became controversial. As a consequence, relationships among occupants of these roles grew unclear, difficult, and sometimes hostile. This applies particularly to many of the professional roles upon which the functioning of social systems depends. From a longer list that would include teachers, the clergy, and various kinds of administrators and managers, I have given emphasis in this chapter to psychiatrists and other mental health professionals, to medical practitioners, and to lawyers. This is in keeping with our focus on the Bristol Mental Health Centre and its goals.

The change can be illustrated by comparing two events in the history of the Centre. As will be discussed in detail later, the problem arose in 1956 of creating a local Board of Directors. The task was accomplished in a few months by joint effort among people in diverse roles, but most particularly by a nucleus that included a psychiatrist, a general practitioner, and a lawyer. In 1970, the Board was faced with another problem that called for cooperation among people in these same roles. The problem – which will also be discussed later – was by its nature more divisive and difficult than the first, but the actions and words of those trying to deal with it revealed that the capacity for cooperation and mutual trust among the psychiatrist, the general practitioner, and the lawyer were not what they had been and, further, that this decrease in capacity for cooperation was related in a major way to changes in how each perceived the other two roles. These perceptions had become much more stereotypic and under the influence of prevailing negative sentiments of the period – in other words, prejudiced. To the occupant of each role, the others were objects of doubt and suspicion. Thus, the interactions in 1970 as compared to those in 1956 appeared more like automatic responses to stereotypes than the interactions of people of good will concerned about solving a local problem that pertained to the common good.

6   The Bristol Centre: staff

Let us now look more closely at the Centre itself, beginning with the staff, and ask what events can further explain the dwindling of goals and goal achievement described in Chapter 4.

Recruitment and maintenance

The basic staff complement during the years of this report was a psychiatrist, a psychologist, and a social worker, plus a secretary-receptionist. Additional persons in one or more of these roles were added for the sake of the research, especially during the first nine years. The total professional staff is shown in Table 3, classified according to roles.

The mean number of professional staff members per year was three, with a range from one to six. The mean rate of turnover was one individual lost and replaced per year. There were, however, long periods when one and even two of the positions were vacant.

It is at once apparent that the Centre was a sand castle, constantly being washed away and rebuilt. This fact accounts for much of the failure to reach goals. The turnover placed serious obstacles in the way of achieving a stable frame of reference, consistently applying scientific thinking, and maintaining priorities.

It was anticipated, of course, in the planning phase and at the initiation of the Centre, that there would be difficulties in finding and holding quality staff. The experience of the provincial government had made this plain. In 1951, despite the beginning of the mental health movement, the orientation and values of private service dominated, and clinical inquiry was primarily in terms of personality psychology rather than social and community psychiatry. Psychobiology was waning and public health psychiatry was for a few enthusiasts only. Then, the Centre was in a rural area isolated from urban professional contacts and stimulation. Thus, the pool upon which it was possible to draw for personnel was exceedingly small. In an effort to meet the situation, the following policies were adopted:

Table 3. *Total professional staff of the Centre during the first twenty-one years.*

Psychiatrists	11
Psychologists	8
Social workers	13
Administrative assistant	1
Total	33

1   The Centre staff should be of the highest quality obtainable. The criteria should include the reputation of the place where a candidate had been trained, the extent of training, and evidence of individual capability as revealed by interview and letters of recommendation.

2   The Centre staff, particularly the director, should be selected from among people with a major commitment to research on the interplay of sociocultural factors and mental illnesses. This was considered central to securing individuals with adequate motivation. Previous work, especially publications, was an important criterion.

3   The Centre staff should, to the full extent possible, be Canadian. This would be in keeping with the location of the Centre and would make the experience favorable to career opportunities and enhance motivation.

4   The positions should involve appointments in the sponsoring university (Cornell). This would create a rational set of role relationships, including clear lines of administrative authority. More important, however, it would mean that the staff were members of a professional group engaged in varying aspects of the same research, all interested in discovery and in developing the field of social and community psychiatry.

5   There should be frequent visits by the Centre staff to the campus of the sponsoring university for conferences, seminars, and informal discussions with colleagues and peers. There should also be frequent visits by professionals (psychiatrists, psychologists, and other social scientists) to the Centre. These exchanges would provide stimulation and resource persons and would affirm the sense of belonging to a company of peers engaged in pioneering a new and growing field.

6   Funds should be provided and time allowed for members of the Centre staff to attend professional meetings according to their wishes and needs. They should also be free to do consulting work and to sit on committees of provincial and national organizations. This would facili-

tate continuing professional contact and development and reduce the sense of isolation.

7   Appointments should be planned in terms of three years. This was not ideal for the Centre's needs, but it seemed a compromise necessary in order to obtain highly capable personnel. The career ladder in psychiatry, psychology, and social work would, it was judged, accommodate a field experience such as the Centre offered for about that length of time. This policy was based on the assumption that work at the Centre would be desirable postresidency and postgraduate training. It was believed that the research goals and the six conditions listed above would give the experience this quality.

8   Salaries should be higher than those obtainable elsewhere for people at this stage in their careers. The aim was to offer some monetary inducement to compensate for the academic isolation and other negative features, but not enough to cause money to be a primary consideration.

9   The expected three-year turnover should be staggered such that the two most senior people would not leave at the same time.

These strategies of selection and reward worked fairly well as long as they were kept in effect. It was, in fact, possible to more than double the staff size in order to meet an increased work load stemming from the combined service and research demands. During the first five years of the Centre's life, it was joined by a total of eight psychiatrists, four psychologists, five social workers and one administrative assistant. The psychiatrists had all undergone a minimum of three years of clinical training, and most had more. Several had additional postgraduate training, and two had research experience in fields directly related to the Centre's goals. All the psychologists held master's degrees, and one was well along toward a Ph.D., which he afterward completed.

Obtaining social workers, however, was a different matter, which later proved to be a camel's nose in the door of our clinical tent. Despite considerable effort, it proved impossible to recruit anybody with a master of social work degree who was interested in the research and willing to do the kind of home visiting and casework described in Chapter 4. The potential candidates who were interviewed all expressed strong commitments to psychotherapy, and such research interest as they had was focused on psychodynamics. Legwork about town and driving about the country were not to their taste.

As an adaptation, the Centre secured the services of a former school teacher who wished to make a career change. He was given a few weeks of orientation through the cooperation of the Maritime School of Social Work and then considerable in-service training and guidance from the

Centre psychiatrists and psychologists. Later, another teacher and an occupational therapist were also recruited and given similar on-the-job training. Thus, a precedent was set in the Centre of improvising with personnel who were not technically qualified. This was the camel. In early years, however, it did not cause trouble, apparently because of the motivation and capabilities of the individuals selected and because of the training and guidance provided.

Taking publication as one indicator of relevant staff ability, it may be noted that ten of the eighteen staff members who came to the Centre during the first five years published before, during, or after their stay at the Centre, and one was a major contributor to *More for the Mind*.[1] Eleven continued in professional careers related to the Centre's goals, and three of these became professors and heads of departments in universities.

In the beginning, staff turnover went somewhat according to plan. The first team (consisting of a psychiatrist, who was also the Centre's director, a second psychiatrist who worked half-time, a psychologist, and the teacher who functioned as a social worker) remained more or less intact until August 1953. This was three years, if the beginning is considered to be September 1, 1950, when the psychiatrists were first employed and began preparatory work. The only changes in the staff complement prior to August 1953 were the departure and replacement of the initial psychologist and the addition of a third psychiatrist for one year.

When the first team left, it was replaced by a second. The break, however, was not total, for the psychologist (who had become Centre director) continued, and the retiring chief psychiatrist nominated his successor. The new team began with two psychiatrists (both full-time), two psychologists, and another teacher functioning as a social worker. An administrative assistant was added and also, for a brief period, a second social worker. This situation remained stable for two years, at which time there was another exodus. The chief psychiatrist left to head a newly created mental health center, and the senior psychologist and the social worker left to pursue further graduate studies. Adjustments were made in which the second psychiatrist became the chief psychiatrist and director of the Centre, aided by the administrative assistant. A new psychiatrist and social worker were added to the staff, and for a six-month period a second psychologist also joined.

Toward the last of these six early years, there was more turnover. The then chief psychiatrist departed, having spent three years at the Centre, and his place was taken by the second psychiatrist; a new psychiatrist came to fill the second position. A third psychiatrist, in a fellowship and training status, was present for three months. A sociologist served as both a researcher and a social worker. This was the situation at the time the Stirling County Study passed administrative responsibility over to a Board of Directors on October 1, 1956. Of the staff then present, however, it turned out that only one, the psychologist, was to remain more than 10 months.

Although there was some orderliness in the way in which these changes were executed, they nevertheless interfered with the stabilization of goal priorities, operational definitions of mental illnesses, and a variety of related activities. They also interfered with the maintenance of relationships with the population of the area, played a prominent part in the failure to complete research projects, and inhibited the development of a training program.

Yet, despite all this, these early years were the period in which the Centre did, in fact, delineate its goals, draw up plans, see an average of over 90 new cases per year, conduct high-quality case management, engage in public education, build bridges to other helping agencies, assist in founding a local mental health society and a second mental health center, triple the size of the area it served, publish two papers, provide opportunities for a masters' and a Ph.D. thesis, and, finally, develop a Board of Directors and turn the responsibility for the Centre over to it.

October 1, 1956, was a critical point in the history of the Centre for two reasons: (1) The provincial and federal component of the Centre's funding was shifted from a research to a service basis; and (2) the local Board of Directors took over control. At the time, there was a staff complement of two psychiatrists, one psychologist, and one social worker. In the next four years, three psychiatrists and four social workers had joined the Centre staff, while four psychiatrists, one psychologist, and five social workers had left. In other words, the total professional staff of the Centre on January 1, 1961, was a single member, a psychiatrist.

These changes were accompanied by internal discord among old and new staff members that was often focused on disagreement about how the service should be operated. At times, the discord reached such extremes that professional individuals went for many months without speaking to one another. On one occasion, this state of affairs was repeated even after a complete turnover in staff.

Meanwhile, the dimensions of the case load to which the Centre was committed by its goals began to emerge from the epidemiological research. The work of the Stirling County Study showed that 20 percent of the adults in the population had some need of treatment for mental illness, whereas only 1–2 percent actually got it from or through the Centre.[2]

Most of the 20 percent who had some need of treatment, however, were not actively seeking help from the Centre, and many were being aided by general practitioners. Nevertheless, they represented a potential case load of considerable magnitude, especially if the outreach goals were to be met.

Those interested in the Centre – the Board, the provincial Mental Health Administration, the Stirling County Study, and the local mental health society – struggled hard for its survival, and in so doing set aside all other considerations. Although staff qualifications and competence were still, in principle, considered important, keeping the Centre open became the first priority. In fact, one Board member went so far as to say "Better a poor psychiatrist than no psychiatrist." The result was diminished attention to the reputation of the place where a staff candidate's training had been received, to achievement of formal qualifications, to interest in the research, and to Canadian citizenship. There was also a lessened effort to find young people for whom the Centre might be an important step in a distinguished career. The Stirling County Study did continue to provide opportunity for the staff to attend meetings outside the province and to visit centers where relevant innovative work was in progress. Under the new fiscal arrangement, however, the Mental Health Administration did not encourage such activities, which blunted their effectiveness as reward strategies for recruitment and retention of staff. As a result, there was a change in staff composition to members for whom academic ties were either threatening or of little importance.

A further consequence of the changes introduced in 1956 was a blurring of the lines of responsibility and authority. The continuing physical presence of the Stirling County Study contributed to this through the Study's powers to control research funds and academic appointments and through its informal influence derived from having created and directed the Centre during the previous years. There was also, however, a great deal of ambiguity regarding the division of responsibility among the Board, the Centre director, and the provincial Mental Health Administration. Even by the early sixties, there was still much policy groping as the provincial Mental Health Administration, successive Centre directors, and the Board sought to define their respective roles. As a consequence, staff members at times felt pulled in different directions and experienced a good deal of discomfort and confusion regarding their tasks.

Another influence was the fact that the practice of giving some hardship pay for working in an "isolated" area was abolished after the transition of 1956. This was the result of a federal policy that stipulated as a condition of funding that the staffs of mental health centers must be paid

Table 4. *Staff joining the Centre between October 1, 1956, and March 31, 1972*

	Male	Female	Total
Psychiatrists	3	0	3
Psychologists	1	3	4
Social workers	4	4	8
Total	8	7	15

Table 5. *Time periods in months when staff positions were unfilled, October 1, 1956, to March 31, 1972*

Staff position	Amount of time position vacant	Percentage of time position vacant
Psychiatrist	0	0
Psychologist	83	45
Social worker	43	23
Psychologist and social worker simultaneously	33	18

according to the provincial civil service scales, even though they were not, in fact, civil servants and did not have the security of civil servants.

From the beginning of 1961, there was a period of comparative stability of staff; this decrease in turnover rate, however, was shortly offset by periods in which there was no person occupying the positions of psychologist or social worker. Staff distribution after 1956 is shown in Table 4, and the periods when staff positions were unfilled are shown in Table 5.

In terms of formal training, most of the staff members after 1956 had fewer advantages then those in the early years. The precedent of accepting technically unqualified people, established at the beginning with the social workers, was extended later to the other positions as well. Concomitant with this acceptance, there was, necessarily, a decline of systematic guidance and in-service training. Of the fifteen staff members who joined the Centre during the later years, a follow-up showed one to have published in a learned medium and one to have gone on to an academic career.

A sentiment expressed in later years by both staff and Board members was that people without advanced degrees or certification, but who had relevant practical experience, were actually better suited to the needs of the local population than those trained in "ivory tower" and "fancy pants" institutions. This sentiment was supported by claims that the un-certified individuals were more down to earth, better able to deal with "real problems," closer to the grass roots, and somehow more basic and democratic.

In favor of this view is the fact that it is entirely possible for gifted people to make up in experience, in reading, and in knowledge of the local area what they lack in formal training, and to perform better than many technically qualified professionals, especially those accustomed to work-ing in urban areas that have a markedly different type of clientele in a markedly different environmental setting from the rural area.

In the case of the Centre, however, actual experience suggests that people without formal qualifications should be employed only when care-ful selection, training, and supervision are possible. General sentiments in favor of the untrained proved to be treacherous. They were, it seemed, in part a rationalization aimed at neutralizing some uneasiness about decid-ing to make do with what was available and so placing at risk the welfare and safety of ill people. They were also, one could infer, an expression of some defensive prejudice on the part of less educated individuals on the Board and on the staff toward the better educated.

Thus it was that the structure of the situation and the accompanying sentiments inclined the Centre to welcome those ideas emerging in the sixties that placed high value on the contributions of paraprofessionals and indigenous workers. The Centre was also favorable to views, many of which were expressed in the school issue described in Chapter 5, that downgraded authority, standards, expertise, and control and emphasized in their place the right of every individual to conduct his job as he saw fit – including the care of patients.

Social processes

Management

Had they possessed administrative skills and training in the theories and principles of organization, the Centre staff might have had a somewhat easier time. Indeed, such technical knowledge might have converted some of what the staff saw as frustrations into interesting, challenging problems. They might have more effectively utilized time, delegated responsibilities, set up methods for decision making, monitored activities, promoted communication, and registered achievement. The applied science of management might have done much to bring about adequate record keeping and helped to remove the staff's sense of limitless burden. The drag on the spirit and energies of the staff occasioned by unfilled positions in the Centre might also have been overcome by a more active and imaginative recruiting program and the development of rewards.

So also, job descriptions, case records, written goal priorities, and guidelines based on the cumulative experience of running the Centre could have made the orientation of new staff more effective and at least somewhat reduced the discontinuities and instability of personnel changes. As it was, the Centre staff, together with the Board and the Mental Health Administration, for the most part approached problems in a here-and-now effort to meet all demands as they arose; they set aside very little time for taking stock, planning the division of work, and delegating tasks. Immediate problems constantly blocked the thinking out of long-run solutions.

There was one period in the early years when the Centre was somewhat better organized than during most of the rest of its existence. This came about as a result of the effort to create a rural mental health center model and lasted for approximately two years. Drawing on Cornell's resources in the fields of management and human relations, the staff tried to clarify standards, roles, and responsibilities. The basic means for ensuring communication, in-service training, mutual learning, and collaboration consisted of regular two- or three-hour staff meetings. There were two of these each week, one focused on patients and one on research. In the former, new cases were reviewed, and the progress of old cases was examined.

Incorporated in this was an organizational feature that was rare for a mental health center, namely the display of a bar chart that depicted work in progress. The objectives of different staff members were shown, and entries reflecting progress were made weekly. The purpose of the chart was to aid coordination and to help members keep track of where they stood amid multiple tasks.

The prevailing philosophy at this time was one that favored mutual respect among staff members of different disciplines and the belief that everyone had important contributions to make. A major tenet was that individuals did best in tasks that they themselves had a share in forming. Staff meetings and one-to-one conferences were occasions when the more knowledgeable staff members could instruct those less experienced and informed and when the members of one discipline could share their perceptions with those of another. Although neither psychology nor psychiatry was considered to be intrinsically superordinate, years in training and years of experience were, and there was a continuous effort toward definition and clarity in the assignment of responsibilities. Obligations to patients were kept uppermost. During part of this twenty-one years, as mentioned earlier, a clinical psychologist was director of the Centre, and for the remainder that role was filled by a psychiatrist.

An egalitarian outlook was also characteristic of the Centre during the later years, but it changed to the more extreme patterns that were then becoming popular, such as those described previously in regard to the Company of Young Canadians. It was assumed that staff members were a company of peers who could divide the work largely according to individual preferences. Such an orientation had potential for challenging each person's sense of responsibility and initiative, and at times it seemed to do this and also to foster a pleasant, socioemotional climate. At other times, however, it seemed to breed discomfort and dissension because of the structureless and unpredictable situations it promoted. These, in turn, provoked angry assertions of authority that were then seen as inconsistent, unfair, and dictatorial.

The fact was that the staff members varied greatly not only in formal qualifications but also in knowledge, experience, energy, concern about patients, willingness to take responsibility, and integrity. They were not, therefore, peers by any relevant definition. Many of them were in need of guidance, information, encouragement toward excellence, help with organizing their priorities, and, at times, being reproved or let go. They received little if any of these when the prevailing sentiments were extremely permissive – allowing each to "do his own thing," and opposing "meritocracy."

In the context of the permissive climate, there appeared to be a belief that somehow the independence of everyone would work out to the greater good of the patients. One can see a possible parallel here to the advocacy of laissez-faire economy as superior to planned economy, and it is worth remarking that members of the Centre staff who would have hotly rejected a laissez-faire economy as unjust and inhumane seemed to have no such reservations about laissez-faire patient care. In actual fact, there were times when concern about patient care was altogether invisible.

Relations with the surrounding society

Social and cultural processes constitute another area in which some knowledge might have reduced the level of staff frustration, heightened interest in the work, and led to greater effectiveness. Just as clinical training helps one to understand rather than react personally to hurtful remarks from patients, so training in social processes can help one to comprehend events and trends that are opposed to his or her aspirations rather than to react personally with frustration, apathy, or anger.

The school issue described in Chapter 5 may be taken as a case in point. The Centre staff rarely, if ever, had a grasp of the schools as a subsystem within a larger social system, nor did they seek to understand the behavior of teachers and school authorities in these terms. Consequently, they did not appreciate why teachers and the school administration were apprehensive about the case-finding efforts of the Centre in the schools. In part, this apprehension came from the belief of school personnel that the inquiry might expose their shortcomings in handling pupils, but it came also from the fear that some children might be labeled by schoolmates as "crazy" or "dumb." The teachers thought that the consequences could include tormenting and teasing by other children and angry reactions from parents against teachers and the administration. Several teachers pointed out that even going for counseling from the regular teaching staff in the high school had at times been a cause of pejorative labeling and social difficulty for students. Both administrators and teachers felt that they could not, however great the need, refer some children to the Centre because of the high risk of adverse reactions among parents, other relatives, and friends. Beyond this fear, the school personnel, though stating their own understanding of the Centre and its purposes, were skeptical that parents generally were ready to accept the principle of a school working directly with an institution that treated "mental illness." There was also some doubt that the mental health professionals really knew as much as many people claimed for them.

The Centre staff could not accept these stigmatizing attitudes as a social reality that could not be changed overnight and that therefore had to be accepted and patiently dealt with while working toward change. Instead, the staff saw stigmatizing attitudes as a grave moral fault for which they blamed individual teachers and school administrators and to which they reacted with outspoken condemnation. Moreover, they interpreted the resistance of teachers to requests for information and other help as indirect expressions of their attitudes toward mental illnesses and did not pause to reflect that perhaps they, the Centre staff, had pushed for too much too quickly and, hence, that the school subsystem was unable to accommodate their requests.

My point is not that there was nothing in the schools that could be altered for the good of the children. It is rather that the Centre's activities in regard to the schools were conducted with the individualistic orientation characteristic of clinicians. They were also conducted blindly, emotionally, and sometimes impulsively. The alternative to this is that they might have been conducted with some appreciation of social processes and so achieved a greater measure of success in bringing about changes beneficial to the children, which is what the staff wanted.

Training in social processes could also, I think, have helped to achieve some burden-relieving utilization of local resources. It could have led, for example, to integration with the hospitals, especially the new general hospital in Bristol when it was being planned. Having a social worker attached to this hospital might have eased some of the demands on the Centre as well as improved the human component in the medical services.[3] Better understanding of societal systems could have made for greater communication and sharing with the family physicians, the welfare subsystem, and the educational subsystem.

What actually happened in the course of time was more or less a disengagement of the Centre from these subsystems. Thus, whereas on the national scene the medical profession (including local doctors) was moving toward group practice and cooperation among physicians, the Centre was, by its disengagement, paradoxically reaching backward toward the individualistic private service model. This was given explicit expression when patients at the Centre were described as the director's "practice" and resentment was expressed at the thought of anyone interfering with his prerogative in this regard.

Efforts were made from time to time by the Stirling County Study and the Mental Health Association to open up opportunities for the staff to learn about social and cultural processes and to visualize the Centre in a setting of social systems. The arranging of staff visits to Cornell, Harvard, and other institutions was part of this, as were seminars offered on the Centre premises. On some of the visits to other institutions, not only the Centre personnel but also the Chairperson of the Board participated.

The most notable and potentially influential conference was one on training in community psychiatry at Arden House, New York, in February 1964. This was one of four "institutes" held across the United States during 1963–64 in order to hammer out a theoretical and operational frame of reference for community psychiatry. The institutes were attended by virtually all the North American leaders in the field and resulted in the publication of the book *Concepts of Community Psychiatry*.[4]

In 1967, one member of the Board made a trip to England and visited numerous mental health and illness services in London and vicinity. He brought back firsthand knowledge of the rapid developments then occurring on the British scene. His report, however, aroused only rather frosty disinterest on the part of the staff.

During this same period, leading professionals were brought to the Centre – such people as Gerald Caplan from Harvard, Henri Collomb from Senegal and France, Milton Mazer from the community program at Martha's Vineyard, and Raymond Prince from Montreal. None of these encounters had any evident impact on the staff, except to elicit complaints that they were exhausting. It may be supposed that this was, in part, because the visits came too late in the training and life experience of the staff members; they were unable to see how to utilize what was laid before them, and for that reason it may have seemed more threatening than helpful.

Opinions and attitudes

Long before the emergence of what has been called the counterculture, there were, of course, numerous individuals who were exceedingly dissatisfied with many of the values and customs in Western society. Lipset has noted that attitudes and sentiments of this kind are characteristic of people in the social sciences and "mind-studying trades."[5] The Centre staff from the beginning contained a number of such rebels, and for some of them the conventions and beliefs of small town and rural life were anathema. This feeling is exemplified by the comment of one sociologist who said, "I was trained to analyze norms, not to uphold them."

The consequence was the occurrence of some staff behavior that implied and some staff remarks that stated, at times with a flavor of contempt, that the local society ought to change its ways and values. These were not well received; they were seen as presumptuous and motivated more by a desire to show off, or by political and economic ideology, than by a desire to cope with mental illnesses in the population.

On the other hand, there were two major patterns of sentiment among the members of the population that made adjustment difficult for the Centre staff, quite aside from adverse reactions to rural values and conventions. One of these was an ambivalent set of feelings toward the "mind-studying trades." The staff members were accorded awe for their supposedly mysterious wisdom, dislike because they might be able to read people's minds, gratitude and appreciation for help given, contempt for being quacks, laughter for being "nuttier than their patients," and resentment because the very presence of the Centre, staffed by strangers, was taken as confirmation of the worst fears some people had about the area and themselves.[6]

This mix of opinions and attitudes is, of course, a manifestation of the emotions roused by mental illnesses. It is met virtually everywhere by those caring for mentally ill persons, and accepting it is part of being a professional. It is, however, especially trying in a small town because of the difficulty of having a social life that is truly separated from one's professional role. Exposure to such emotions is therefore almost constant. One of the best clinicians the Centre was able to recruit left because, as he said, "I thought the community did not trust me."

The second major pattern of sentiment that unsettled many staff members was the tendency of the people to disparage themselves. Although there were many people who had high regard for themselves, their neighbors, and their way of life, their self-regard was more than matched by the negative orientation of others. Few of the staff, when arriving as newcomers to the area, were prepared for the persistence with which they were taken aside and told that virtually everything "hereabouts" was inferior and hopeless. This unbalanced condemnation fell upon the whole range of human endeavor from economics and politics to education and recreation, very often with an emphasis on deficient ethical and intellectual behavior of leaders and neighbors.

The impact on staff members was twofold. First, to the extent that they accepted the picture as truth, it confirmed some of the urban and academic prejudices they had brought with them and added new distortions. As a result, some staff members acquired a distaste for the county and a desire to leave. Second, even some of those who were able to see the disparagement as distortion and to appreciate the resources of the area nevertheless soon became saddened and exasperated. They found, time and again, that it slowed up cooperative projects designed to achieve some of the Centre's innovative goals. The possibility of joint action among local people was apt to be denigrated by the local people themselves, and expressions of altruism might be treated with silence or probed for hidden selfish motives. The climate of feeling was one that discouraged not only effort but also concern about excellence. As one individual said, "the trouble with people here is they'll pick up an old rusty nail when the job calls for a new brass screw." Thus, with a single sentence, he both exhibited disparagement and described one of its consequences: When you disparage everything, nothing matters.

Disparagement was far from being prevalent all the time or among all people, or drawn by every target equally. It was common enough, however, that it is not an accident that the main research paper produced by the

Centre staff was one that focused on disparaging attitudes.[7] In my opinion, furthermore, the general tendency to disparage was a background factor of some importance in the previously described school issue. It encouraged too ready acceptance of hostile and negative statements.

At the time the Centre opened, people by and large considered city life to be better than country life. This was especially noticeable among the young. A few of the older generation, including some who had been away and come back, preferred a "slowly paced, traditional style of life exemplified by physical labor in a natural environment; . . . absence of intense drives toward achievement, yet a strong desire for independence and personal integrity; development of . . . warm communal relatedness and immediate gratifications; . . . satisfaction with stable interpersonal relationships and currently meaningful activities."[8]

By the mid-sixties, "urban sprawl" had come into disrepute, along with much else in Western culture, and there were many persons, especially young people, who sought new meaning for life in Stirling County and other such areas. The county is, in fact, a region of great natural beauty, providing possibilities for closeness to sea, fields, and forest. Handcrafts, folkways, farming, fishing, working in the woods, and opportunities for providing human services are all there, together with group belonging, cooperative projects, or, on the other hand, freedom for independence and social detachment. It is a place where one need not be overwhelmed by competition and the demands of material values and where one can find numerous resources for that self-realization, harmony with nature, and spiritual development claimed by many as the most desirable objective in life.

Social crisis and the Centre

As was discussed earlier in this chapter, the relationship between the staff of the Centre and the Bristol school system was a troubled one. It grew worse in the latter part of the sixties. When, in January 1970, tension began building toward a crisis among the population of the town over the dismissing of the teacher (see Chapter 5), Centre staff members entered the dispute on the side opposed to the school administration. Their participation took shape in letters to the press and to officials, public speeches, appearances on TV, and membership in the citizens' committee. Vigorous action along these lines went on through most of the period of tension and then increased as the crisis began to recede. Various members of the Centre's Board of Directors, of the Mental Health Association, and of the Stirling County Study tried to persuade those involved that the Centre's role should be nonpartisan and cooling and that it should try to help the participants find a framework for a rational and just solution. The director of the Centre said little in reply to these overtures except to state that in the last eleven years the leaders of the Board, the Mental Health Association, and the Stirling County Study had "done nothing," whereas he had now "crashed in and produced substantial changes of great benefit to children in the community." He shortly afterward resigned from his Harvard appointment and from cooperation with the Stirling County Study.[9]

It was about this time, in the spring of 1970, that the local doctors' concerns for the way patients were handled by the Centre staff came to the fore. The nature of their complaints were summarized in Chapter 4 and need not be repeated here.

We can, however, enlarge a little on some of the complicating factors. The chairperson of the school board was a physician, and both he and most of the other doctors took a dim view of the manner in which the Centre had been participating in the school issue. Furthermore, the superintendent of the schools was also the chairman of the hospital board, and the director maintained that criticism emanating from the medical subsystem was in reality the result of his actions on the school issue. He also said that as a matter of principle he would have nothing to do with an organization (the hospital) that was chaired by the superintendent. Suggestions continued to be made by the doctors, by members of the Mental Health Association, by members of the Centre Board, and by members of the Stirling County Study that one way or another urged getting together in a spirit of mutual sympathy and understanding in order to examine the problem of patient care. These were, however, all rejected on the grounds that the proposals were not what they purported to be but were, in fact, aimed at discrediting and ousting the staff from the Centre.

Concluding note

This review of the Centre's staffing history puts into the foreground the problems of recruiting and holding personnel – a theme that ran through the mental hospital and mental hygiene movements and that still runs through the mental health movement. Although strategies that prevailed during the early years of the Centre were to some extent successful, they were later given up. The turnover of staff members interfered in a major way with the continuity of activities and the achievement of goals.

That interference was enhanced by those attributes of the mental illness field that were summarized in Chapter 2 as barriers one and three –

heterogeneity and lack of an accepted frame of reference. Individuals from different backgrounds brought to the Centre different frames of reference, different interests, and different emphasis in their work. Every change of face, therefore, meant a period of disequilibrium followed by a new equilibrium that was never the same as the previous one. Objectives were added, goals were modified, and activities were altered. Priorities, especially, tended to shift. This must always happen to some extent in human enterprises, but the porous and amorphous character of the mental illness field maximized the fluctuations.

Although staff turnover affected all the goals and activities of the Centre, it did not do so equally. Thus, diagnosis and treatment procedures were somewhat less affected than others. This is perhaps because they constituted, at least during the fifties, an area in which there was an approximation of clinically uniform ideas. This consensus should not be overstated, but it did seem to hold true when a new staff member had about the same amount of training as his or her predecessor. By and large, the methods for treating people with psychotic conditions, anxiety, depression, and brain syndromes did not alter drastically with changes in personnel – and, as we have seen in Chapter 4, these conditions made up the greater part of the Centre's actual case load.

The situation was different with regard to personality disorders, sociopathic behavior, and social adjustment problems. With these conditions, there was much more variation among therapists in manner of patient handling, and there was less certainty regarding the division of work and responsibility among psychiatrists, psychologists, and social workers.

Consultation and referral patterns were quite variable from one staff member to another, and they were sometimes marked with rather strong feelings. For example, staff members differed notably about what kinds of patients should be accepted for treatment and what kinds should be referred back to the family physician or elsewhere.

The innovative goals outlined in Chapter 4 regarding the development of area resources, research, training, and university affiliation flagged the most. This was despite the fact that the Centre was itself originally an innovative effort. The negative trend seemed to be in part due to personnel changes – there was never time to bring these projects to fruition – and in part due to the advent of uninterested staff members. It is important to add, even if it anticipates subsequent chapters, that the innovative goals and activities were also those that were least understood by members of the Centre's Board of Directors, by the Mental Health Administration, and by the population at large. In fact, after the formation of the Centre's

Board of Directors in 1956, the only strong support for these goals came from the Stirling County Study.

The perception of being overloaded with cases was a staff characteristic throughout the period covered by this report. There were times when the belief was undoubtedly well founded, as for instance during the months when all work had to be handled by a single psychiatrist. It is also true that silting with frequently returning chronic patients was a serious problem. Mostly, however, the time actually devoted to patient care by staff members was not excessive by medical standards. In later years, at any rate, they worked from nine to five for the most part and did not spend nearly as many hours per week in seeing patients as did the family physicians of the area. The Centre was always closed on weekends, and it was rare for staff members to see patients on Saturday, Sunday, or in the evening. The complaints about case overload, therefore, did not represent what was actually happening, and it is necessary to seek an explanation elsewhere.

The talk about a large case load seems to have been in some degree the result of faulty management and in some degree an expression of the staff members' fears that they would not be able to cope with what was expected of them. What was expected is contained in the description of the universal public service model outlined in Chapter 5 which had been growing in the consciousness of Canadians during the years following World War II. A major threshold was crossed when the Royal Commission on Health Services issued its report in 1964: "What the Commission recommends is that . . . as a nation we now take the necessary legislative, organizational and financial decisions to make all the fruits of the health sciences available to our residents without hindrance of any kind."[10]

In the Bristol area, universal services were advocated by the Mental Health Administration, the Mental Health Association, and the Stirling County Study. In the meantime, everyday clinical experience, not to mention the epidemiological findings of the Stirling County Study, made it evident that making "mental health" care available to all residents of the area served by the Centre was an impossibility. The staff members were under pressure, therefore, to achieve the unachievable.

Apprehension about their ability to cope may also have had another dimension for some staff members, namely, a sense of insufficient training, skills, and experience. Consultation and referral, research and evaluation, preventive measures, the development of area resources, and the provision of training, together with university affiliation, could each or all have been seen as beyond an individual's capacity and therefore as involving high risk of failure and ridicule. For those whose clinical training had been short and incomplete, the situation must have seemed that much worse.

If these interpretations are correct, they can add something to our understanding of why the Centre pulled away from the hospitals and doctors of the area and moved from the universal public service model toward a pattern of independent private services. Case load, in fact, was explicitly stated as a reason for rejecting affiliation with the general hospitals. The diminishing of connections with the doctors was not so explained, but analysis of the Centre's records show doctors to have been the main channel by which new cases arrived at the door.

There is still another possible factor. In discussing types of medical practice and role strains across Canada, Blishen says, "The lack of observation of the solo practitioner's professional conduct by his peers means that there is a minimum of professional control over the quality of the services he provides, particularly outside the hospital." Blishen adds that referrals and consultations increase "the degree of observability of his professional activities by his peers . . . thereby creating pressure upon him to maintain high standards of medical care."[11]

If the tendency of the Centre staff to separate itself from the medical subsystem can be seen as an effort toward the easing of perceived threats, how then does one explain the Centre's often simultaneous emphasis on prevention?

One explanation is that these moves served the double function of seeming to conform to expectations and at the same time providing an excuse for not seeing patients. For example, one Centre director outlined his policies by saying:

Rather drastic limitations were imposed upon the provision of treatment of well established illness by physical methods . . . The Clinic's activities are now oriented toward the initiation, first, of a service of front-line psychiatry to contain maladjustment and abnormalities in early stages and, secondly, to the development of services of a preventive nature by the provision of family counselling, marriage guidance, child guidance and community education in mental health.[12]

Although it was impossible, given the small size of the Centre's staff and the population of the geographic area, to "contain maladjustment and abnormalities in early stages" and to provide "family counselling, marriage guidance, and child guidance" to all who needed it, one could put in motion activities of this sort without having to be accountable for results. Considering the circumstances under which the Centre (and virtually all other such services) operated, there was little likelihood that there would ever be any kind of real administrative assessment of what proportion of human problems in the geographic area were actually being reached and to what degree primary and secondary prevention were actually being accomplished. The Lord Ronald syndrome, in other words, could operate as a defense – even as a cover under which to hide idleness.

All this occurred against the background of a period when psychiatry, like medicine generally, was developing resources that brought both increased power to help and increased power to harm. It was also a time when, according to Blishen, the patient load on all doctors in Canada was increasing at the annual rate of 4.4 percent.

The practicing physician today [1969] must cope with a medical and non-medical environment in which the application of his skills is made more and more difficult as both these interacting contexts change at an increasing rate. This difficulty creates a growing possibility of error and sanction by his professional peers.[13]

A major contributor to the stresses experienced by the staff of the Centre was the approach and ultimate establishment of Medical Services Insurance in Nova Scotia on April 1, 1969. This change was heralded and followed by much discussion and worry regarding two issues: (1) how much supervision and interference there would be by the government in matters of patient care; and (2) how much checking up and control there would be of "preventive" activities. Virtually all physicians in the province were concerned about the first of these, and professionals in the mental health centers were, in addition, concerned about the second.

These issues created for the staff a sense of being surrounded and advanced upon by exceedingly threatening events. A feeling of powerlessness must have occurred and been added to their long-standing perception that too much was expected of them. It is possible that foundations were thus laid for reactions of anger, revolt, and the desire to break out of the powerlessness. Revolt was also encouraged, of course, by the values that became widespread in the sixties regarding the evils of "the establishment."

Stress and reaction to stress, however, are only part of the picture. Although escape from anxiety and other unpleasant feelings engendered by stressful circumstances is a motivating force in human behavior, consideration must also be given to positive and active (as contrasted to reactive) thrust – termed *spontaneity* by Meyer.[14] Seen from this view, staff efforts to escape from a threatening dilemma were mixed with striving toward objectives such as recognition, self-realization, aggrandizement, and power. Much of what happened during the school-issue period can be understood in such terms. As Blackmer has said:

The ideology of the rebellion is a confused one, a crazy-quilt of many strands, not always in harmony with each other and lacking a clear, well-defined pattern or center. Yet the fact of its existence in many parts of the world excites an irresistible urge to discover a common meaning in it all, to find some central unifying, all-encompassing explanation, to be able to say "at bottom" it is this or that. The causes, in reality, are multiple and interrelated.[15]

The most obvious policy and administrative lesson to be derived from a consideration of the Centre staff is that excessive stresses should not be allowed to build up in a system. There is, however, another lesson of equal importance: the desirability of providing recognition and reward to a staff for good patient care. It is evident now that the stresses experienced by the Centre staff were offset very little by such rewards. The structure of the situation and the various activities of the Mental Health Administration, the Board, the Mental Health Association, and the Stirling County Study failed to create them. The staff members were the unintended victims of inadequate training, poor selection, weak management, and insufficient rewards.

7　The Bristol Centre: Board of Directors

The Centre's Board of Directors exemplifies one of the early attempts to fulfill the ideal of community control of a "mental health" service. It was an ideal which was to be highly regarded in subsequent years partly because of the practical necessity of making services conform more adequately to the needs of the people served and partly because of a philosophy that called for local autonomy and individual rights. In the mid-fifties, a Board that would in some degree represent the population of the area served was seen primarily as a way to secure protection against both the self-serving tendencies of the professions and the unilateral decisions of a distant, monolithic, government agency.

The Board's charge

The Board did not have a charge in the formal sense of a written document given to it by some person or committee in authority. There was, however, an apparent consensus in 1956 among a group of local leaders, the Centre staff, the provincial Mental Health Administration and the Stirling County Study. This may be summarized as follows:

The Board of Directors is to be responsible for running the Centre within the general framework of law, government regulations, and government policies. Specific components of this framework include: acting as employers of the Centre's staff, with powers to hire, fire, and discipline; applying for and receiving annual grants from the provincial and federal governments through the provincial Mental Health Administration; raising additional funds from other sources; managing the total budget; developing policies geared to the needs of the people of the area; working out plans for equitable geographic distribution of services among the districts that make up the service area; and working cooperatively with all local helping agencies, both governmental and voluntary, so as to improve their impact on the mental health of the population; to provide mental health services to patients in the municipal hospitals; to provide consultation service for the physicians practising in the area; to accumulate knowledge and analyse information

118

obtained by the Centre as a basis for research into local problems; and to provide opportunity for observation, instruction and research in mental health matters.[1]

The group that developed the charge did so within the framework of expectations about how other relevant groups and agencies would function. These expectations can be summarized as follows:

The responsibility of the provincial Mental Health Administration was to include helping coordinate the Centre with all other mental health services of the province; managing the dispersal of available government funds so that expenditures would conform to policies, regulations, and the best interests of the taxpayers; and, finally, seeing that proper technical and professional standards of patient care were maintained. These functions were to be performed by the Administration from its position as a division of the Department of Public Health.

The provincial Mental Health Association and the local Mental Health Society were visualized as aiding the Centre through public education regarding mental health in general and the Centre's program in particular; through raising supplemental funds; and through supplying volunteer help as needed.

The physicians practicing in the area were expected to supply guidance by being members of the Board. It was thought that the best mechanism for their participation would be the nomination of representatives by the medical associations in each county served by the Centre.

The Stirling County Study was asked to stand by with such help, funds, and advice as the Board might need after taking over the Centre. The Study was to remain in control of research.

Cooperation among these several agencies and associations was seen as essential if the Board were to function properly. Plans were therefore made to include on the Board physicians and nominees from the Mental Health Society and to have ex-officio positions occupied by the administrator of the Mental Health Administration, the district public health officer, the head of the Department of Psychiatry at Dalhousie University, and myself as head of the Stirling County Study.

For other members of the Board, emphasis was on balanced representation from three counties, with special reference to local (town and municipal) governments and to people expected to have a particular interest in human services such as the clergy.

Origins of the Board

When the Centre was introduced to the people of its area in 1951, it came as a foreign body into a complex of preexisting social subsystems and sentiments. There was, at the time, little concern with, or even awareness of, mental health and mental illnesses in the areas. Indeed, despite the interest of doctors, teachers, and certain others, many people looked on the Centre as both anomalous and superfluous. Nevertheless, we of the Stirling County Study hoped that the Centre would evolve from its foreign-body status into a functioning component of the area's social structure. Our background of experience and research in applied anthropology gave shape to this aspiration, and also to a general strategy for bringing about its accomplishment.

After the Centre had been in existence for a year or so, it was evident that there were a wide range of specific sentiments in the population and that these could be grouped in terms of three categories: positive, indifferent, and negative.[2]

Those people expressing positive sentiments saw the Centre as beneficial, a resource that ought to be fully utilized. Doctors, clergy, and some teachers expressed these opinions, together with those patients who had benefited from the Centre and their families.

Indifference – that is, little awareness of the Centre and less interest – was by far the most widespread state of mind. People with such views, or, more properly, lack of views, were regarded by the Stirling County Study as an asset because they did not press the budding service with demands for which it was not yet prepared, were not opposed to it, and constituted a potential target for educational effort as the Centre became ready.

Negative sentiments were, of course, those hostile to the Centre, and several reasons for them were apparent. First, it is generally to be expected that virtually any innovation will disturb the customary roles of some individuals and the activities of some subsystems in a society, and these individuals and subsystems are prone to resist and counterattack, overtly or covertly. In the case of a psychiatric center established in a small town and rural area, the people most likely to perceive themselves as threatened are those whose roles involve some aspects of practical psychotherapy and counseling. Doctors, clergy, and school personnel are of this number, together with the informal "gatekeeper" whose advice is sought when individuals have personal and emotional problems. Thus, some of those who perceived their roles to be threatened were the same persons who favored and even sponsored the creation of the Centre. This fact highlights the complexity of the valences acting upon the functioning of an organization such as the Centre. A second type of negative sentiment is one I mentioned in the previous chapter, namely, the common antagonism people feel toward the "mind-studying trades," even when professing the opposite.[3] Third, in gaining support from one segment of a geo-graphically defined population, one always runs the risk of also acquiring that segment's enemies. Bonds with a political party or a religious group can obviously have such consequences, but, more subtly, so can connec-tions having to do with leadership rivalries and antagonisms between fac-tions and kinship networks. It is probably impossible to avoid this kind of entanglement altogether, but the Study tried to have the Centre act and be recognized as nonpartisan in every way. The policy was to emulate the philosophy of a Bristol town barber who, when asked how he was going to vote in a coming election, replied, "I always keep my mouth shut on politics because hair grows on Tories and Grits alike." A fourth type of hostility may be summed up by the word *prejudice,* which was directed at categories of persons among the Centre and Stirling County Study per-sonnel. This included antipathy toward individuals from urban areas who had advanced educations, but it also focused on staff members because they were American, British, Jewish, black, from upper Canada, or from Quebec. For the most part, prejudices of this kind were not strong, but on occasion they did give some trouble. The policy of the Centre and the Study was to proceed as if they did not exist, and in general this worked.

The Study endeavored to have the Centre move slowly in matters of community action and to concentrate on meeting felt needs, such as treat-ing the mentally ill persons referred by doctors. It was thought important that time be allowed for the spread and digestion of information and for the formation of opinion according to the normal processes of the society. Despite some ambitious leaps ahead that caused trouble (for instance, trying to screen all the school children and analyze what teachers were doing) and some talking about prevention that may have been premature, the Centre did, on the whole, demonstrate a service that came to be val-ued by doctors and by the patients and their families. Table 2 (in Chapter 4) points this out by showing that on the local scene, after the doctors, the main sources of referral were self, family, and friends. As a result, bridges were built between the Centre and various subsystems of the society, and the realization that the Centre existed not only expanded but became more and more colored with positive feelings.[4]

Once a favorable aura had been created, people began to wonder what else besides direct care of the mentally ill the Centre might take on, and they came forward with suggestions and requests. Various area organiza-tions, such as churches and service clubs, began drawing personnel from the Centre into their activities, and individuals and groups began showing spontaneous interest in how they might help the Centre. Thus, opportunities were created for the Centre staff to begin pursuing the array of goals outlined in Chapter 4.

The situation was at this stage in 1954 and 1955 when the question of changing the Centre's administrative structure had to be considered. The immediate reason for this was a federal representative's recommendation that the government portion of the funding be shifted from a research to a service basis. He pointed out that the change would give the Centre permanent status and eliminate the need for periodic reapplications for grants, as was required in the case of all research funding. He further suggested that this change need not make any significant difference in the conduct of research at the Centre because, as things stood, the government grant was actually supporting the service component of the enterprise, whereas private funds (from the Carnegie Corporation of New York and the Milbank Memorial Fund) were financing the data collection and analysis.

The prospect of changing the administrative structure generated discussion about the possibility of having a Board of Directors, but it is difficult to say now precisely where the proposal had its origin. Examples in school boards and hospital boards had, of course, long existed. As applied to mental illness services, the idea was newer but was nonetheless in the air, and was certainly in the mind of the administrator of the Mental Health Administration. In 1954, the Scientific Committee of the Nova Scotia Society for Mental Hygiene (by then a division of the Canadian Mental Health Association) issued a report in which it recommended that there be "community participation, e.g., boards, auxiliaries, etc.,"[5] and there were parallel discussions going forward in New England.[6]

The reason my colleagues and I in the Stirling County Study favored community control was in large measure due to previous research experiences. These had included studying the administrative problems of Eskimo and American Indian groups and also of Japanese-Americans relocated during World War II.[7] Such studies had led us to conclude that, by and large, people use services better when they participate in their management than when the services are simply provided by some outside authority. This view was reinforced by the works of Holmberg, Opler, and Whyte[8] and by studies from the Department of Rural Sociology at Cornell, which had for many years been active in rural development.[9]

Moreover, the social science studies that we had conducted in Stirling County itself, beginning in 1948, indicated that although there were trends toward disintegration of social structure, there were also numerous strengths in the social systems of the county and rising trends that ran counter to disintegration. Severe disintegration, our research showed, was confined to a few small clusters of population, and these were matched by an opposite pole composed of one or two well-integrated groups of 300 to 400 people. These groups easily merited the term *community* more or less in keeping with the ideal model to be discussed in Chapter 8. The other population clusters of the county, which amounted to some 90 in all and which included the town of Bristol, lay mostly in a middle ground between these poles.[10]

It seemed to me that the mental health Centre might well exert an influence that would foster integration and reintegration and that a board derived from a number of local towns and villages might be one step in this direction. Our initial effort was experimental in its orientation. We wanted to see what a board, and also the Centre as a whole, might do to foster social integration where it was needed in pursuit of goals that concerned the public good. This was congruent with one of the Stirling County Study's long-range goals, namely, exploring the feasibility of primary prevention for some kinds of mental illnesses. Looking back now, it seems apparent that the experimental orientation faded somewhat in the course of time as I and other members of the Stirling County Study became caught up in the struggle for the Centre's survival. We did not do the repeated stocktaking expected of observers and analysts, or at least did not do it often and thoroughly enough. We allowed hopes and wishes to outrun judgment and so shared in the overconfidence in community competence which has characterized much of the mental health movement.

In regard to a board of directors, the Fundy Mental Health Centre, which was being established at Wolfville in 1955, set an example through planning to include one as part of its organization. This was probably derived in part from the Mental Health Administration and from the influence of the Acadia Institute (an affiliate of Acadia University), which was a prime mover in establishing the Fundy Centre. There was also some input from the Stirling County Study inasmuch as several of its staff served as advisors to the Fundy group. When the director of the Bristol Centre left to become the first director of the Fundy Centre, one of the conditions he laid down in accepting the post was that there be a board of directors drawn from the population of the area served.[11]

Discussion regarding the roles and functions of a Board for the Bristol Centre began in 1955, among the Centre staff, other members of the Stirling County Study, and the Mental Health Administration. We in the Study expressed our view that the time was ripe for transferring the Centre to local control and thus achieving our goal of having it become an integral part of the area's social system.

The Mental Health Administration was not in the beginning convinced about the desirability of a board. For a time, it had contemplated having the Nova Scotia Hospital play a central role in supplying services to all parts of the province. An advantage of this was that the hospital's location in the Halifax–Dartmouth metropolitan area would likely make recruitment and maintenance of staff easier and that services to the rest of the province could be supplied on an intermittent or rotating basis. The Nova Scotia Hospital itself, however, had for years been chronically short of the staff required to operate its intramural services. At the time the Centre was established, for example, it lacked three psychiatrists in its table of organization.[12]

The Centre might have been managed directly by the Mental Health Administration, but it too was understaffed. In this case, the trouble was not a matter of vacant positions but rather one of a lack of positions. The Scientific Committee of the Nova Scotia Society for Mental Hygiene called the situation at the Mental Health Administration "impossible" and recommended that two new positions be created: a clinical assistant and an administrative assistant to the administrator. It further stated that "the function of the Clinical Assistant . . . be for the development and *supervision of adequate treatment services* and *training programs* in the provincial mental health services. He should be highly qualified and experienced and acceptable for appointment to the teaching staff of Dalhousie University."[13]

This, in effect, would have meant operating the Centre directly from the administrator's office and opened the way for drawing Dalhousie into the program. The government, however, did not authorize the recommended positions, and so the idea came to nothing. In fact, the administrator had a major new duty added to his tasks: Inspector of Humane and Penal Institutions.[14]

Some other alternative, therefore, had to be chosen. The minutes of the discussions that occurred in 1955 between the head of the Mental Health Administration, the Centre staff, and the Stirling County Study show that after some initial hesitation, the administrator accepted the principle of a local board, saying that although he had reservations, he thought the arrangements at the Fundy Centre might be used as a model. Following this agreement, the discussion took up the topics of location, form of control, and implementation of the Board. These did not appear in advance to be questions of great difficulty, yet the first two turned out to have serious, long-lasting negative effects on the Centre and its Board.

The question of location became an issue when the administrator astounded the group by saying that the Centre should be moved from Bristol to Harwich. His arguments were that the latter would be more appropriate in terms of geography and population and that, in addition, the people of Harwich were considerably more interested in having the Centre than were the people of Bristol. Although the first of these points had some substance, the second was at best moot.

The Stirling County Study was opposed to a change of location because that would violate its commitments to the people of the County and because it would effectively divorce the clinical services from the epidemiological research. The cumulative nature of the cultural, social, and psychiatric data that was being collected, beginning as far back as 1948, made the research nontransferable at that time to a new area. The Study and the Centre staff felt that, in suggesting the change, the Mental Health Administration was proposing to go back on agreements it had made with the Study in 1950.

When the possibility of a change in location was brought to the attention of the local citizens who were supporters of the Centre, there was an outpouring of letters and telegrams to the provincial government that resulted in a statement from the minister of health that the Centre would not be shifted.

To this day, I am not sure whether the Mental Health Administration and its parent, the Department of Public Health, really contemplated moving the Centre to Harwich. An alternative possibility is that the proposal was intended as a basis for bargaining for more services to the latter. Another is that the Administration was vacillating because of pressures from within the government, very likely fanned by requests from Harwich. Or the proposal of moving the Centre may have been a balloon sent up to see how strong the wind was blowing, and from what direction.

In any event, if bargaining were intended, it worked; the Centre did greatly increase attention to Harwich, a matter that can be regarded as constructive from the viewpoint of that county. Also on the plus side is the fact that the threat of moving the Centre galvanized the interest of Bristol leaders, and this was likely helpful in the formation of the Board.

On the other hand, the increased attention to Harwich by the Centre was given at a cost to the efforts to reach the original goals in Stirling County. Also a negative result was the abrasive relationship that developed between the Mental Health Administration, on the one hand, and the Bristol leaders, the Centre staff, and the Stirling County Study, on the other. The abrasions were soon healed on the surface, but remained apparent as feelings of uncertainty, if not mistrust, on the part of the Centre and its local supporters. The episode played a part in the development of sentiments that were more adverse than collaborative.

Discussion about control moved from initial hesitancy on the part of the Administration to the placement of a heavy load of responsibility on the shoulders of the proposed Board, as indicated in the summary of the charge. The administrator became attracted to the idea of having a local organization that would relieve his understaffed office of local management tasks. He expressed concern, however, that the Board members be strongly committed and competent and that there be genuine support from the population of the area.

In line with these thoughts, the administrator asked the Stirling County Study not to make a sharp break with its administrative responsibilities, but rather to keep a hand on things until he could see how well the Board functioned. He also asked that in order to demonstrate commitment and community support the Board raise a certain amount of funding from local sources. He pointed out that in the case of the Fundy Centre, its Board was very successful in raising local money.

The Stirling County Study agreed to stand by during the transition and also agreed that it was appropriate for the Board to raise money through voluntary contributions from the area served. The Study thought, however, that it would be unrealistic to expect a level of contribution from the Centre's geographic area that would compare with that obtainable for the Fundy Centre, the latter being situated in an exceptionally wealthy part of the province. The Study suggested that during the time of transition it would continue as in the past to make contributions to the operating expenses of the Centre. In order that there not be a precipitous drop in the financial resources, the Study offered to provide $5,000 per year for three years, beginning July 1, 1956. This was considered to be "on behalf of" the people of Stirling County. The expectation was that at the end of three years the provincial (including federal) contributions would have increased and the Board would be in a position to take charge of raising the additional funds necessary.

In agreeing to delegate authority to the proposed Board, the Mental Health Administration made clear that it would retain control over all monies coming from provincial and federal sources. Thus, the Board would have to submit its budget for approval each year. This seemed at the time entirely reasonable, and yet, because most money would inevitably come from the government, there was implicit in the arrangement a power of veto that could be used to invalidate practically all authority delegated to the Board. This possibility turned into a reality of coercive threats that were exceedingly troublesome in subsequent years, and it called into question the whole idea of the Board having any real authority.

Discussion about arrangements for research and training also raised questions of control, because the administrator seemed reluctant to let the Board have full say in such matters, even though none of the relevant funds then in view were to come by way of the provincial government. In contradistinction to the federal representative, who had suggested that research should proceed much as in the past, the administrator stated that teaching and research must henceforth be severely restricted in favor of service.

This led the director of the Centre to prepare a memorandum[15] for the administrator and local leaders in which the following points were made:

1   That up to that time the provincial government had been unable to staff two of its other three clinics outside the Halifax area. The reason the Bristol Centre had been able to maintain a staff was that the research opportunity was attractive to well-qualified psychiatrists.

2   That the research was an aid to the service activities. The store of basic material on file enabled the Centre staff to help patients far more quickly than would otherwise have been possible.

3   That the kind of research done at the Centre and proposed for the future would rely almost entirely for data on material that a good clinic would collect routinely in any case.

4   That the work already done had given the Centre a measure of recognition and prestige among sources of research money. This would ease the way for future grants.

5   That if the research deteriorated, the Centre would lose its attractiveness to funding sources. This would mean deterioration in operations due to inability to attract and hold competent staff. Thus, quality of service would decline concomitantly, and the Centre could well cease to exist.

The administrator eventually agreed in principle that research should be a component in the future activities of the Centre but was apparently never very contented to have done so. In later years, he often expressed negative views toward research at the Centre to both Centre staff and members of the Board, although not to the members of the the Stirling County Study. It would appear that he thought of research and service as two separate categories of activity that should be organized, funded, and administered independently, out of fear that otherwise the services might be harmed. At the same time, he was a person who in principle strongly favored research, as is attested not only by his public statements but also by the grants approved under his administration.

The pivotal point is that even administrators who favor research do not necessarily see it as yielding results that they themselves might utilize here and now to change services and policy. On the contrary, they are likely to erect walls against any such possibility. The advantages they see are much more in terms of publication in learned journals and some reflected prestige for the administration that sponsored the work. The model in mind seems to be something like launching a spacecraft: The administrators want the work to be a success and contribute to human knowledge and well-being, but they also want all this to occur out in space, not in their offices.[16]

It would be unfair, however, to picture administrators as mainly focused on avoiding trouble to themselves. Many are greatly concerned with avoiding harm to programs in which they deeply believe. The administrator with whom we dealt during the formation of the Board and afterward was, in my view, misguided in his overprotectiveness of the services, but this sprang from an enormous and lifelong dedication to the relief of human suffering among mentally ill persons and to its replacement with enjoyment of life. In pursuing this he willingly stepped, on a number of occasions, into the path of serious oncoming trouble.

Both the administrator and the Stirling County Study saw implementation of the Board as something that should be done gradually. The Study undertook to begin discussions with members of the Bristol Mental Health Association in order to form an advisory group that would take major responsibility for creating a board. These conversations resulted in a letter that was sent by the director of the Centre to a selection of local leaders.[17]

Dear Mr.   :

The staff of the Bristol Mental Health Centre and members of the Cornell Research Programme have, for some months, felt the need for a closer working liaison with the people living within the area we are serving. Several recent and proposed changes in the nature and extent of these services have made the need for such a liaison more acute. One of these changes which has had a large effect on the distribution of our services is the extension of service to Harwich County. Since the 26th of January 1956, we have been holding a Clinic once a week in Harwich town. There are indications that in the future, this amount of time will have to be increased. In a less formal manner, we have also begun to see patients from Kingston County as they are referred to us. This expansion of service has given rise to problems of time distribution and we feel we need the help of a local Advisory Board to reach an adequate solution to this problem.

The forthcoming change-over from a service-research basis for the Center to one that is more strictly service oriented will take place on the 1st of October of this year. This proposed change again makes the need for a local advisory group more pressing, since the clinic orientation will be primarily one of service to the counties of Stirling and Harwich and we feel that the individuals within these counties should have a voice in helping make the best use of what service is available.

For these reasons I am writing to you as a person who is well suited to represent the viewpoint of persons in your county or community and to ask if you would be willing to serve as a member of a temporary Advisory Board. The major functions of this Board would be to determine the necessary formal organization of an Advisory Board and to determine what representation a more permanent Advisory Board should consist of in order to best act as a voice for all the areas which need to be served by the Centre. It is planned that within the next year or so, a permanent Board of Directors will result from the planning of an Advisory Board.

I hope that you will be willing to serve in this capacity. A letter from you, expressing your wishes, would be greatly appreciated.

The first meeting of the temporary Advisory Board will be held in the near future.

Sincerely,

The first meeting took place on March 21, 1956. those present included four local leaders, of whom one was the warden of the municipality in which the Centre was located; the two psychiatrists from the Centre; one of the divisional public health officers (representing the provincial Mental Health Administration); and a member of the Stirling County Study, making eight in all. An Advisory Board was formally constituted, a general practitioner (one of the local leaders) was elected president, and the director of the Centre was chosen as secretary. After agreement that there should be monthly meetings, discussion turned to ways and means for making the Advisory Board representative. It was proposed that there should be three members from Harwich County, including one physician; three members from Kingston County, including one physician; and eight members from Stirling County, including one physician; representatives from the provincial Mental Health Administration, the Centre, and the Stirling County Study were also included. Five meetings of the Advisory Board were held, the last being on August 22. By this time, agreement had been reached on the organization, functions, and membership of a permanent board. A voluntary organization called the Western Nova Scotia Mental Health Group was incorporated on the 29th of August. This body was empowered to provide the Centre with a Board of Directors. All members of the temporary Advisory Board became members of the new board, and the physician who had been president of the advisory group became chairperson. The director of the Centre continued ex officio as the secretary, and a treasurer was employed on a part-time basis.

Thus, the Board contained twelve local members and four ex-officio members, two from the Department of Public Health, one from Dalhousie and one from Cornell. The secretary and the treasurer were not members. The first meeting of the Board of Directors took place on the 17th of October 1956.

Board achievements

The portions of the Board's charge in which it was most successful were those that pertained to "applying for and receiving annual grants from the provincial and federal governments through the provincial Mental Health Administration; raising additional funds from other sources; managing the total budget;" and working out "equitable geographic distribution of services."

The Board worked closely with the director of the Centre, generally accepting his suggestions, and it made annual representations to the Mental Health Administration with regard to the Centre's monetary needs. It was also successful in securing annual appropriations from town and municipal governments in the geographic area. The task of raising money from voluntary contributions was by mutual agreement delegated to the Bristol branch of Mental Health Canada (the Canadian Mental Health Association), which in time replaced the original Bristol Mental Health Society. Because of a major overlapping of membership, particularly among leaders, much of the fund raising by the Mental Health Association was in fact done by individuals who were also members of the Centre's Board. The Mental Health Association eventually provided the Centre with a house to serve as its premises. To do this, the local association, with the help of the provincial association, secured a mortgage and then raised money annually by voluntary subscription to pay the interest and reduce the debt. This arrangement replaced rent money that had previously been supplied by the Stirling County Study.

The Board, through committees, looked after such things as building maintenance, care of the grounds, and housekeeping. Matters of public relations were handled jointly with the Mental Health Association. Through this, and through informal ties that members had in many different parts of the area, the Board was successful in helping the Centre achieve an established position in the social systems of which it had become a part.

The success of the Board in fund raising and related activities was due not only to much effort and good judgment but also to the fact that some of the members had experience with similar tasks in other organizations. The work was, in short, along familiar lines in a setting of well-recognized cultural patterns. These advantages of clarity and familiarity, however, did not apply to many of the other Board charges.

Two major problems faced the Board shortly after its inception. One of these was recruiting Centre staff, and the other was the expansion of services to cover a larger population and geographic area. With regard to the recruitment problem, since the Mental Health Administration appeared unable to assist, the Board asked the Stirling County Study to take charge. The Study agreed to do so, in line with the commitments it had made at the time the plans for the Board were being formed.

The geographic problem was tackled by the Board itself, and many hours were devoted to assessing needs and trying to determine the most equitable allocation of the available manpower. The outcome was the creation in 1961 of a separate Centre at Harwich with its own Board and staff and a geographic area that included a neighboring county. The Bristol Centre retained Kingston and most of Stirling County, but it reorganized, adopted a new constitution, and took a new name – the Bristol–Kingston Mental Health Service Board.

The period from early 1961 through 1963 was a time when the Board was particularly vigorous. It strove hard to achieve appropriate representation in its membership, to define its authority and functions, and to establish its autonomy in relation to the Mental Health Administration. The new constitution of 1961 stipulated that the membership would be as follows:

From Stirling County

6 members from the Bristol Branch of the Canadian Mental Health
  Association
1 representative from the Protestant clergy
1 representative from the Catholic clergy
1 representative from the medical association
1 representative from the Bristol town council
1 representative from the municipal council of Windsor (a component
  of Stirling County)
1 representative from the municipal council of St. Malo (a component
  of Stirling County)

From Kingston County

6 representatives from the Kingston Branch of the Canadian Mental
  Health Association
1 representative from the Protestant clergy
1 representative from the medical association

1 representative from the town council of Kingston
1 representative from the town council of Valleyton
1 representative from the town council of Belcentre

The ex-officio members were shorn of their voting privileges but were retained as "advisory members." These were the mental health administrator, public health officers, and "a representative to be appointed by the President of Cornell University," in other words, a member of the Stirling County Study.

Two new advisory members were added, the director of the Centre and the executive director of the Nova Scotia division of the Canadian Mental Health Association. The head of the Department of Psychiatry of Dalhousie had resigned in the meantime, and no one from that university was specified in the new bylaws.

Thus, there were, in all, twenty-four local members divided equally between the two counties, plus six advisory members.

Unfulfilled expectations

In terms of the charge, the Board did not do well with regard to running the Centre, exercizing the powers to hire, fire, and discipline the staff, developing policies to meet the needs of the people of the area, working cooperatively with the local helping agencies, guiding the Centre's accumulation of knowledge and analysis of information as a basis for research into local problems, or providing the opportunity for observation, instruction, and research in mental health matters.

Even some of the Board's accomplishments were not without a negative side. The raising of money, for example, was an achievement of importance, but a consequence of it was that the activity became very largely an end in itself, divorced from Centre goals and from long-range planning. Instead, the Board behaved somewhat like a team competing in an athletic event, determined to bring back a trophy for which it would be admired in the home area. In the meantime, policy and operational matters went unattended.

The most serious of the unfulfilled expectations was the lack of Board control over the staff. The Board was wholly unable to exert a mending influence when services faltered, could not guide the staff toward meeting community needs when these were overlooked, and did not restrain the staff from community action which the majority of the Board members thought unwise. I have already presented illustrations of these difficulties in Chapters 4, 5, and 6, so it will, perhaps, be sufficient merely to remind the reader of four examples:

1   The development of distance between the Centre staff and the medical subsystem of the area, despite federal, provincial, and the Board's own policies calling for cooperation and effective working relationships

2   The development of distance between the Centre staff and most of the other human services in the area, a drift opposite to the policy described in the charge as "working cooperatively with all local helping agencies . . . so as to improve their impact on the mental health of the population"

3   The unilateral decision by the Centre staff to make social action a top priority and to implement this by joining one side, and employing advocacy and confrontation, in a dispute and crisis about the schools

4   The failure of the Centre staff to respond to complaints from physicians regarding the way patients were being treated

The complex of factors responsible for the Board's functioning as it did came through a wide array of sociocultural and psychological processes. A selection of the more important of these will be reviewed and discussed in the next two chapters.

8 The Bristol Centre: community participation

The Stirling County Study, as the reader may recall, hoped to see the Centre transformed from a foreign body introduced into Bristol to a component of the society in the area. A Board of Directors was conceived to be one of the main channels of this transformation inasmuch as it would open up a means for community participation in the work of the Centre.[1]

The notion of *community* as a basic subdivision of society played a major role in the thinking of the Stirling County Study personnel because of the nature of the research. Community was the unit in terms of which variations in sociocultural disintegration were assessed and compared across the county. These studies showed that there were over ninety clusters of people, each designated by a place name, among which the county's population of 20,000 was divided. The clusters varied in size from about a dozen individuals to one town of approximately 3,000 – namely, Bristol.

The field studies also showed that the degree of integration and disintegration varied considerably from one place-name cluster to another. In some few, the process of disintegration had gone so far as to make it inappropriate to apply the term community in almost any sense. For the greater part of the county, however, processes of integration and reintegration were quite evidently also at work, and some communities gave evidence of being exceedingly well integrated and functionally cohesive.[2]

In planning for the Centre, we in the Study thought first of links with Bristol, the community in which the service was physically located, and then of links with the other larger towns and villages. The dangers to community participation imposed by disintegrative trends were recognized, but it seemed to us on the whole that in these towns and villages integration had the upper hand. Our expectation was that this state of affairs would continue and possibly increase. It also seemed possible that success by local people in the task of taking over and managing the Centre would strengthen trends toward integration.

Unanticipated, however, was the arrival from North America at large of the behaviors and sentiments characteristic of the sixties and described in Chapter 5. Many of these can be interpreted as expressions of deepening sociocultural disintegration. They caused a widening crevasse between popular notions of what communities are and changing social realities. We must understand these differences if we are to understand both the achievements of the Centre's Board of Directors and its failure to fulfill the expectations of the Mental Health Administration, the Stirling County Study, and some of the local leaders who participated in its founding.

The community concept

The word *community,* like mental illness, encompasses so many disparate meanings that two people can employ it and believe they are talking about the same thing when they are actually speaking of quite different matters. The New Oxford Dictionary gives seventeen definitions, including such oddities as an "ordinary occurrence" and a "common prostitute." The meanings in more current use include the following (abridged and in part paraphrased):

1   The quality or state of having social intercourse, fellowship
2   A body of individuals having equal rights or rank
3   People with certain characteristics in common such as occupation or religion, but not shared by the others among whom they live, such as the "medical community" or the "Protestant community"
4   A body of people living in the same locality
5   A body of people organized into a political or social unit, which can range from a village to a nation
6   An equivalent of the word "public"
7   A group of people living together for religious or political reasons; for example, a community of monks
8   Gregarious animals such as bees

The dictionary also quotes a reference by Galen to a person who had a "community of ulcers."

Although the word is usually employed without indication as to which of the above meanings is intended, it is often evident that the idea in mind is a mix of several of them, plus some others. Thus, the *ideal community* has geographic boundaries, is self-sufficient and self-determining, has democratic decision-making processes, and is characterized by feelings and beliefs that emphasize civic responsibility, pride, caring for the rights and needs of others, and "we-feeling" or sense of identification. The historic New England town, with its town meeting, is sometimes mentioned as a paradigm.

In searching for this model in real life, we must take note of five points having to do with social structure and five having to do with sentiments. All ten may be considered a mixture of realities, perceptions, and sentiments that constitute obstacles to community functioning, somewhat comparable to the four barriers to progress in the mental illness field outlined in Chapter 2. The existence of all fourteen unhappily suggests that the words *community mental health* often stand for a bog of misconceptions and misperceptions.

The five points in regard to social structure are the following:

1. In a modern North American "community," the *boundaries* are difficult to define because they are often different for different purposes. Ecological, economic, political, and census boundaries rarely coincide. Neither do the boundaries of health, welfare, and school districts. The lines drawn for any one of these purposes may enclose several of the others, or cut one or more in two. These are not trivial problems because they influence the flow and coherence of information, the capacity of agencies to cooperate, the effectiveness of leadership, the ability of people to feel that they are part of a community, and the creation of public support.

2. A very large part of the *economic and political decision making* that affects a town takes place elsewhere. Many of the stores, restaurants, and other businesses are not, as they were years ago, locally owned but are, instead, components of chains; and industrial plants are often units in a complex structure of holding companies. It happens, therefore, that in places hundreds or perhaps thousands of miles away from a town, decisions are made to open a new shopping plaza or to close a factory with little regard to local effects; and the local citizens can do nothing about them. The case is similar in education and in health and welfare programs. Policies about the content of school curricula or the qualifications of teachers, for example, are made by professionals in capital cities distant from the local scene. This is not to imply necessarily that poor service results, but only that there is much about it that is beyond a community's reach.

Because of decision making at a distance, local governments are often weak. For instance, Vidich and Bensman observe that "Decisions which are made locally tend to consist of approving the requirements of administrative or state laws. In short, the program and policies of local political bodies are determined largely by acceptance of grants-in-aid offered them."[3]

Because of town needs, the state, provincial, or federal grants are not usually a genuine option. They must be accepted, and once accepted local freedom of choice is enclosed by the conditions of the grant. Furthermore, as Tocqueville observed many years ago, the situation is often ambiguous because it is very difficult when dealing with governments to distinguish their advice from their commands.[4] Schottland states that local people have trouble in performing their functions because their "planning mechanisms are not equipped to cope adequately with the impact of the various Federal programs."[5]

Vidich and Bensman point out that "The complexity of organizing political support; the necessity for historical, legal and technological knowledge in defining an issue clearly; the lack of knowledge of procedure, the lack of time – all these factors lead to inaction."[6] Consequently, as Warren observes, "Although the actual legal scope of local governmental authority is fairly limited, the village and town officials do not even make use of what authority does exist for the pursuing of common activities on the local level. There results a 'political paralysis.' "[7]

3. *Voluntary organizations* have similar disabilities. This applies especially to those organizations that are concerned with the common good and focus on schools, hospitals, mental health, and welfare. For instance, Sower and his colleagues, writing about health councils, say that they tend to be powerless, incapable of long-range planning, and lacking in public support. The people who hold office discover that it is difficult to find successors, and much of the organization's energy goes to a struggle for survival.[8] Commenting on voluntary health-oriented groups more generally, Warren describes them as showing duplication of effort, lack of coordination, and "lack of adaptation to the specific needs of the local community."[9]

One must wonder why they can be characterized in this way when the voluntary groups are composed of local persons. The characterization arises from the fact that many of the people who hold positions of influence in towns have a primary, often unspoken, allegiance to individuals and groups outside. These *hidden constituencies* are composed of the officials above the local managers of banks, accounting firms, and chain-stores. It is common policy for companies to encourage participation by employees in prestigeful voluntary organizations but at the same time to discourage involvement in controversy that might antagonize a segment of actual or potential customers. This has a dampening effect on the mobilization of decisive action. It makes for passivity, appeasement, and lack of commitment and of moral leadership.

4. *Geographic mobility* produces a turnover in a sizable proportion of a town's population every few years, a process that undermines the leadership structure and makes policies inconsistent. Geographic mobility also

affects general-public as well as leader participation in community affairs. This is because those who see themselves as transient or who use the town only as a "bedroom" often do not feel it "worthwhile to get involved."

5. Participation by citizens who are not geographically mobile is also limited. As a result, the affairs of a town rest in the hands of a mosaic of *special interest groups* who singly (and even when taken all together) may actually constitute only a small proportion of the population. Special interest does not necessarily mean a selfish interest – it may indeed be entirely altruistic – but it does mean a narrow base as far as representation of the views of the inhabitants are concerned.

Let us consider for a moment the concept of *representation*. The members of hospital boards, mental health center boards, and so forth, are commonly said to "represent the clients" or "the people of the community." Yet it is often doubtful that they really do this. They are, as a rule, self-selected in terms of their personal interests, and if they have any disposition to be active, it is in furthering what they are convinced the public ought to have rather than what the majority actually wants. As Kolb has said, referring to the situation in the United States:

There has not been a single directive from any federal or state agency willing to define the nature of representation. Nor have I heard a single community leader, or elective representative stand and define it. It has surprised me that all of these groups, while speaking of community control, have been unwilling to define how one gets representative groups from a community.[10]

The reason is evident – they do not know how.

In considering these various matters, it is important not to lose sight of the fact that towns vary considerably, some being more and others less like the ideal community. As Warren sums it up:

Presumably, communities vary in the extent to which they are merely "junctions" for regional and national networks of goods, services, and institutional behavior patterns and control, with little locally initiated and locally determined action, on the one hand; or, on the other hand, the extent to which they are strong locality groups with the bulk of their activities, though following regional and national cultural patterns in varying degrees, nevertheless initiated, determined, and directed from within the community itself.[11]

Community program planning, therefore, is exceedingly risky unless one knows the recent history of the community in question and its level of functioning and competence.

The five points discussed so far have to do with the dimension of social structure. Parallel with social structure is the dimension of shared sentiments,[12] about which the following five points should be noted:

1. In many towns today a cluster of sentiments exist that may be summed up by the word *inertia*. For example, despite the reputation Americans have for being "joiners," Wright and Hyman concluded in 1958 that they are only weakly so and that there are marked differences in joining that depend on socioeconomic class. Utilizing data from two national surveys, they reported that 64 percent of Americans belonged to no voluntary association, 20 percent to one organization, and 16 percent to two or more organizations. Quoting from the report:

The pattern of voluntary association membership among different occupational levels indicates even less participation among blue collar workers than had been noted in previous local studies. For example, from 68 to 87 percent of the blue collar workers belong to no organization (not counting union membership), in contrast to 59 percent of the white collar workers and 47 percent of the businessmen and professionals.[13]

People who are engaged in action to correct harmful defects in human services have frequently commented on the resistance they encounter. Thus, Hunter speaks of the "unwilling public" and notes that leaders will not budge because of various apprehensions such as the likelihood that taxes will be increased, that those in need of the services are unorganized and silent, and that the majority of the people between those two groups are apathetic.[14] In such situations, welfare workers who see the needs and speak out for them find that they have little support at any level.

Inertia, to some degree, is an essential component in the functioning of any society. Without it the system would be hypersensitive to every passing stimulus and liable to disaster from too many reactions in too many different directions. Inertia, therefore, works up to a point to counteract sociocultural disintegration. Like many compensating mechanisms, however, it can progress to such extremes as to become destructive.

2. A second cluster of sentiments, one already met in Chapter 6, may be labeled *self-disparagement*. This consists of denigration of the locality and its people together with the feeling that nothing much good happens or can happen there. Most things worthwhile are thought to happen elsewhere, especially in prestigeful urban centers. "Our town" is seen as a "backwash," the "sticks," or a "booney" from which everyone with brains and ability gets out as fast as he or she can. There are, of course, people who hold contrary views, but in many communities disparagement reaches such proportions as to make the society seem to be suffering from severe emotional depression. This is not to say that individual inhabitants are clinically depressed in unusual numbers, but rather that their shared sentiments make the town as a whole very like a depressed individual who has a gloomy, self-mistrusting outlook, difficulty in concentrating on problems, and difficulty in reaching decisions for action. An overlay of

defensive town boosting that may also be present does not negate the underlying sentiment.

3. Another sentiment has to do with the great importance attached to at least superficially *maintaining good relations* among all people who have face-to-face contact. This short-range pervasive sentiment takes precedence over behaviors that might otherwise flow from moral principles and long-range concern for the common good. "Don't rock the boat" is a directive of extraordinary force. Vidich and Bensman noticed in the conduct of local government that

> no member irrevocably commits himself on an issue, and hence does not alienate himself from the other members of the board with whom he must deal from month to month and in his daily living on a friendly basis. These dynamics explain the lengthy and poorly directed discussion which occupies the time of the board.[15]

The dynamics also explain an observable phenomenon in the governance of many communities and voluntary organizations that might be called the "dry cleaner syndrome." It consists of dealing with routine and easy matters on the premises but shipping away difficult decisions for someone else to take care of. Difficult decisions are those about which public opinion is either divided or generally hostile. These arise because any governing group, however local, gains knowledge that is different from that possessed by its public. As a consequence, the leaders find at times that what they believe to be the right decision is one that will excite disfavor. A common ploy, therefore, is to have the decision made by some higher authority outside the area. In this way the onus can be taken from their shoulders and blame attached to the "bureaucrats," "the government," the national headquarters of a voluntary association, or the still more remote "they" who are at the bottom of so many appalling decisions.

The habit of shipping ugly problems out of town undermines self-determination and autonomy inasmuch as it invites and strengthens outside intervention in local affairs. The higher authorities of the provincial, state, and federal governments are not willing to play only the role of villain in the eyes of a community. If they are directly or indirectly pressed to make unpopular decisions on difficult issues, they are bound to insist on having a say about the factors involved in the origins and consequences of these issues. The proponents of local participant democracy in health and other helping services must find a solution to this dilemma because it is evident that they cannot have it both ways – independence for comfortable decisions and dependence for the nasty ones.

The sentiment against rocking the boat is not confined to leaders who need a political following but is communitywide. People feel that the best treatment for trouble and troublemakers is avoidance. Up to a point, of course, this makes good sense and promotes social cohesiveness. Carried beyond this, however, it means that people are reluctant to come forward and defend others whom they know to be exposed to injustice or bad care. As a result, chronic inefficiencies of services and malignant social processes such as graft, robbery, and vandalism are allowed to take root and grow.

In discussing the desire to avoid trouble in interpersonal relationships, I have not intended to overlook the existence of hostile factions and long-standing feuds in many towns. These, however, like racial prejudice, are most often expressed in economic- and political-power moves rather than in open confrontations. They are also deplored by the population generally, who feel a strong desire to prevent their growth.

4. Another important point is that many community sentiments have spread from urban areas.[16] This *diffusion* is an element in the disparagement complex because the city does in many ways look down on smaller places. The press, the radio, and the television that reach the country are almost entirely urban in orientation and emotional tone. In addition, modern transportation and the disposition to geographic mobility bring town and rural dwellers to cities for varying lengths of time and, similarly, bring city relatives and holidaymakers to the country. As a result, town and country people are exposed to what goes on in cities and the world more generally.

To illustrate the spread of urban sentiments, let us look briefly at Robert Merton's description of what he calls *cosmopolitan* and *local influentials*. The point of relevance is that cosmopolitan sentiments, which are to a large extent at variance with community ideals, appear to have been increasing in rural areas, whereas those of the local influentials, which are in keeping with the popular notion of community, have been diminishing. Merton describes and compares the two systems of sentiment as follows:

In the process of making their mark [the local] influentials have become thoroughly adapted to the community and dubious of the possibility of doing as well elsewhere. From the vantage point of his seventy years, a local judge reports his sense of full incorporation in the community: "I wouldn't think of leaving Rovere. The people here are very good, very responsive. They like me and I'm grateful to God for the feeling that the people in Rovere trust me and look up to me as their guide and leader."

The cosmopolitan influentials are very different:

Not only are they relative newcomers; they do not feel themselves rooted in the town. Having characteristically lived elsewhere, they feel that Rovere, "a pleasant enough town," is only one of many. They are also aware, through actual experience, that they can advance their careers in other communities. They do not, consequently, look upon Rovere as comprising the outermost limits of a secure and satisfactory existence.

Local influentials attach great importance to knowing many people and to having

all manner of personal contacts which enable them to establish themselves when they need political, business, and other support. Influentials in this group act on the explicit assumption that they can be locally prominent and influential by lining up enough people who know them and are hence willing to help them as well as be helped by them.

The cosmopolitan influentials, on the other hand, are more selective: "It is not *how many* people they know but the *kind of* people they know that counts." In short, the "locals seek to enter into manifold networks of personal relations, whereas the cosmopolitans, *on the same status level,* explicitly limit the range of these relations." Both kinds of influentials are inclined to join voluntary organizations, but the type of participation is different:

Cosmopolitans are concerned with associations primarily because of the activities of these organizations. They are means for extending or exhibiting their skills and knowledge. Locals are primarily interested in associations, not for their activities, but because these provide a means for extending personal relationships.[17]

In summarizing, Merton says that "the composition influential has a following because *he knows;* the local influential because *he understands."* But let us note that both are somewhat paralyzed as activists in town affairs: the cosmopolitan because of his hidden constituents outside the town, and the local influential because of his need to avoid ruffled interpersonal relationships within the town.

5. The final point about shared sentiments pertains to the *we-feeling* or sense of belonging together. This exists in some measure in many towns and villages, but it is often weak as a basis for action because of such other sentiments as inertia and not rocking the boat. These anticohesive trends are strengthened by the uncertainties that accompany rapid social change and by the consequent feelings of heightened suspicion and mistrust.

The popular notion of community becomes less appropriate as one moves up the scale of size from villages and towns to cities and metropolitan areas. It is probably unnecessary to argue this point at any length because it is well recognized that most of the large urban areas in North America suffer from a trend toward social disorganization that is expressed in administrative inefficiency, class conflict, ethnic and racial difficulties, poverty, public debt, strikes, crime, and the like.

Nevertheless, there have been some attempts to apply the community model to geographically defined sections of cities and to signal this application by calling them neighborhoods. Both health and mental health centers have been created and their policies set under the influence of such assumptions, particularly with reference to participation and control by neighborhood people. The "catchment" areas of these centers have usually included many different neighborhoods in all of which the kind of problems just described for towns are present at higher levels of complexity and magnitude.

In sum, the community model is a risky one because it often fails to match actual conditions. It has, moreover, a dangerous appeal due to what is in many of us a strong nostalgic desire to believe in its validity. Such a belief satisfies numerous longings that arise in reaction to the troubles of contemporary society. As a result, we often assume the model's truth when we would be better advised to doubt and examine it carefully.

Community characteristics of the Bristol Centre's Board of Directors

Against the background of the preceding section, we may now take a more detailed look at the Board of Directors of the Bristol Mental Health Centre. We shall begin with some of its numerical characteristics and their patterns of change across time.[18] The reader will have little difficulty in recognizing some of these as quantitative demonstrations of deviations from the ideal model of community functioning. The data reflect such problems as geographical mobility, representation, inertia, and cosmopolitan influence.

The Advisory Board lasted seven months and held five meetings. The expected number of local members was fourteen; the number actually achieved was eleven. Of these, two dropped out and two others were not strong participants; hence, the number of active Advisory Board members[19] came to seven, or 50 percent of the expected number. All members were males. In geographic terms, five were from Stirling County and two were from Harwich County. No one responded from Kingston. The occupational distribution is shown in Table 6. The same chairperson presided throughout this short period.

The first permanent board, the Western Nova Scotia Mental Health Group (for convenience, designated hereafter as WG), lasted four years and three months.[20] The expected number of members was again fourteen, and again this figure was never achieved. Over the whole period, the modal number of members was eleven, or 79 percent of that expected.

Turnover in WG membership was considerable. Nine members carried

Table 6. *Occupations of active and total members of the Advisory Board*

	All members	Active members
Management	3	2
Physicians and dentists	3	1
Teachers (including administration)	2	1
Farmer	1	1
Attorney	1	1
Reporter	1	1
Total	11	7

Table 7. *Length of service of members of the Western Nova Scotia Mental Health Group*

	Number of members
Serving one year or less	7
Serving two years	2
Serving three years	2
Serving the duration of the Board	8
Total	19

over from the Advisory Board, and ten others were added at different times, giving a cumulative total of nineteen members over the life of the Board. Nine of these, however, left before the end of the period. The various reasons for leaving the Board and the number of persons involved in each category were as follows: health, one; shift of interest, three; moved away from the area, five. The length of service contributed by members is shown in Table 7.

It is apparent that of the nineteen people who were members of the Board, seven, or almost 40 percent, served less than a year. Of these seven, six were among the ten newcomers who had not been part of the Advisory Board. The WG, we may conclude, had significant problems with membership turnover and with short-term service during the same

Table 8. *Occupations of members of the Western Nova Scotia*
Mental Health Group

	All members	Active members
Management	5	3
Teachers (including administration)	3	2
Physicians and dentists	3	2
Clergy	2	0
Housewife	1	0
Attorney	1	1
Farmer	1	1
Reporter	1	1
Unknown	2	0
Total	19	10

years that these same problems were major difficulties in the Centre staff. The Board was, however, stabilized by a core group of active members.

Defined in terms of general interest, evident participation, and service on the WG for at least two years, the active members numbered ten out of the total of nineteen who joined. The fact that two of these dropped out about the midpoint and were replaced by two others means that at any given point in time the active number was eight, or 57 percent of the expected complement of fourteen. The cumulative total of ten active members was 53 percent of the total (nineteen) who joined the WG. The modal attendance at meetings was seven, with a range from four to ten.

The ten active members in the WG included eight of those carried over from the Advisory Board, seven of whom had been active members of that group. As we have reported earlier, the president of the Advisory Board became chairperson of the WG and continued in that position throughout the period. In sum, then, the core of the WG was mainly a continuation of the active members of the Advisory Board, and only a small amount of success was achieved in developing the Board beyond this.

The occupational profile of the WG is shown in Table 8. This profile very much resembles that of the Advisory Board (see Table 6). In terms of sex, there were two women among those who served on the WG, one of whom was active.

Table 9. *Organizational sources of members of the Western Nova Scotia Mental Health Group*

	All members	Active members
Mental health associations (including the Bristol Mental Health Society)	11	7
Municipal councils	2	1
Clergy	2	0
Physicians	1	1
Unknown affiliations	3	1
Total	19	10

To achieve some kind of representation, it was planned to draw Board members from various organizations or subsystems of the region. The results of this for the WG are shown in Table 9. As is evident for both total and active members of the WG, the mental health associations of the two counties were the main sources of Board members.

The second permanent Board, the Bristol–Kingston Mental Health Board (for convenience, designated hereafter as BB), came into existence in January 1961 and lasted beyond the concluding date of the study (March 31, 1972). The time period covered is therefore eleven years and three months.

The expected number of members was twenty-four, but, again, this was never achieved. If we define a member as anyone so mentioned in the Board's minutes, then the maximum number at any time was twenty-one, whereas the mode was twenty. If we exclude nominal members such as the doctors who virtually never attended, the modal membership drops to eighteen. In these terms, the BB was always 25 percent short of its expected complement.

Only two of the seven active members of the Advisory Board carried over into the BB, and one of these dropped out shortly afterward. There was thus, at this time, a marked attentuation of the original founders of the Board. Part of this loss was due to the fact that one of the original seven went to the Harwich Board. Of the eight active members of the WG who were present when it dissolved, two went to Harwich, and four of the remaining six did not participate in the BB. One of the four moved away from the area, and the other three apparently had a shift of interest. Those grouped under "shift of interest" had all served for more than four years

Table 10. *Length of service of members of the Bristol–Kingston Mental Health Services Board*

Length of service	Members who dropped out	Members on the Board March 31, 1972
1 year, more or less	14	10
2 years	8	0
3 years	1	3
4 years	2	0
5 years	2	0
6 years	1	0
7 years	2	1
8 years	0	1
9 years	0	3
11 years	0	2
Total	30	20

and may well have felt that the Centre was on its feet and that they had accomplished what they had set out to do. Altogether, then, only one active member of the Advisory Board and one active member of the WG participated to any significant extent in the BB.

The cumulative membership of the BB – that is, all members joining the Board during the time we covered it – was fifty. Thirty of these (60 percent) left the Board before the end of the eleven years, and twenty (40 percent) were still members at the end of March 1972. The length of service given by both groups is shown in Table 10. It is apparent that almost half of those who came and went served on the Board for about a year, some a little more and some less. Twenty-two, or 73 percent, remained on the Board for less than two years. If we consider service of more than two years as the minimum necessary to contribute effectively, then only eight of the thirty "transient" members qualify. The members of the BB at the end of our time period show a very similar pattern. Ten out of twenty had, as of that time, served only about a year. On the other hand, there is a group of seven members who had served between seven and eleven years.

The apparent reasons for leaving the Board are shown in Table 11. It would seem from this that geographic mobility was a major cause of people leaving the Board. The next strongest association was that of being a delegate from a town or municipal government.

The existence of eight members who served between three and seven

Table 11. *Apparent reasons members dropped out of the Bristol–Kingston Mental Health Services Board*

	Number of members
Left the area	10
Representatives of local government[a]	8
Health	3
Physicians[b]	3
Retirement	1
Shift of interest	1
Joined Centre staff[c]	1
Unknown	3
Total	30

[a] The dropping out of representatives from local government was in part related to changes resulting from town and municipal elections and in part to rotation of assignments.
[b] The withdrawal of all physicians from active participation on the Board has been noted in the text.
[c] Staff members were ineligible for a place on the Board.

years points to a group of potentially active members among those who served on the Board but left before the end of the eleven years. When these are assessed in terms of meeting attendance and participation, five can be considered active members. Including those active members who served two years would raise this number to seven. In sum, of the thirty Board members who came and went during the first eleven years of the BB, between 17 and 23 percent were active members of the Board.

With regard to those who composed the Board at our cutoff date in 1972, ten individuals (50 percent) had served between three and eleven years. Eight of these can be classified as active, which is 40 percent of the actual Board members, but only 33 percent of the expected Board complement of 24. This may be compared to the 57 percent figure of the WG and 50 percent for the Advisory Board.

These tabulations do some injustice to those who were newcomers to the Board in 1972, a number of whom were active participants, but it seems appropriate to omit them from the core group of members because they had not had time to gain even rudimentary familiarity with the Centre and its problems. This is in keeping with our treatment of the people who served less than two years before dropping out; some of these were also active participants during their short tenure.

Table 12. *Occupations of members of the Bristol–Kingston Mental Health Services Board*

	Members who dropped out	Members remaining in 1972
Clergy	9	3
Management	4	6
Teachers (including administration)	4	4
Physicians[a]	3	2
Housewives	3	0
Attorneys	2	1
Blue-collar workers	2	0
Farmer	1	0
Public health nurse	1	0
Social worker	1	0
Pharmacist	0	1
Reporter	0	1
Accountant	0	1
Unknown	0	1
Total	30	20

[a] As mentioned in the text, even though physicians were carried in the Board's records as members, their membership must be considered nominal because of nonattendance at meetings.

Looking at occupations, Table 12 indicates no great difference between the members who left the Board and those who were on it in 1972. A comparison of active members with the total membership is shown in Table 13. This suggests that through the years most of the active members of the BB came from management and teaching, few from the clergy, and none at all from among physicians.

Out of the total of fifty members, nine were women, of whom four have been classified as active. Among the forty-one men, ten were active. One might speculate, therefore, that although women were less likely to become members of the BB than were men, a higher proportion of those who did were active. The chair was occupied by four individuals during the course of the eleven years, one of whom was a woman.

Sorting the active members from all the boards into cosmopolitan and local influentials resulted in the tabulations presented in Table 14,[21] which indicates that whereas the Advisory Board and the WG were dominated by local influentials, the BB came to be more strongly under the

Table 13. *Occupations of active and all members of the Bristol–Kingston Mental Health Services Board*

	All members	Active members
Clergy	12	1
Management	10	5
Teachers (including administration)	8	3
Physicians	5	0
Housewives	3	1
Attorneys	3	1
Blue-collar workers	2	0
Reporter	1	1
Farmer	1	1
Accountant	1	0
Public health nurse	1	1
Social worker	1	0
Pharmacist	1	0
Unknown	1	0
Total	50	14

Table 14. *Active Board members divided into locals and cosmopolitans*

Active members	Locals	Cosmopolitans	Locals (%)
Advisory Board	5	2	71
WG	8	2	80
BB, members who left the Board	3	4	43
BB, members remaining in 1972	3	5	38

influence of cosmopolitans. The fact that the six ex-officio and advisory members of the Board and the staff, who attended the meetings, were all cosmopolitans makes it plain that through time the Centre grew to be an organization in which local influentials were numerically weak. A similar trend with regard to influence is illustrated by the five chairpersons who served the Board between 1956 and 1972. The sequence was local, cosmopolitan, local, cosmopolitan, cosmopolitan. In terms of years, most of the first half of the period between 1956 and 1972 was chaired by locals, whereas most of the second half was chaired by cosmopolitans. This was

Table 15. *Organizational sources of active and all members of the Bristol–Kingston Mental Health Services Board*

Organizations or Subsystems	All members	Active members
Mental health associations	29	13
Clergy[a]	5	0
Physicians[b]	3	0
Local governments[c]	13	1
Total	50	14

[a] Altogether, 12 clergy served on the Board, but only five of these did so as representatives of the clergy. The others represented one or another of the mental health associations.
[b] Five physicians were nominally on the Board at one time or another, but only three were considered to be representing the doctors. One of the others represented a local government, and one a mental health association.
[c] One of those grouped under mental health associations also represented a local government for a short period of time.

not the kind of leadership that had been visualized when the Board was established.

Because cosmopolitans are in general more task oriented than local influentials, it might have been expected that they would seek some kind of action when the issue of proper patient care was raised. There was, however, an obstacle to their doing so, namely that almost every one of them had a hidden constituency or reference group by which he guided much of his behavior, including that of getting on the Board in the first place. The effect of these hidden constituencies was to motivate such members to avoid controversy at all costs, as noted in the previous section on the community concept.

The organizations and subsystems of the geographic area that were sponsors of the BB members are shown in Table 15. It is plain that the BB was in general dominated by members of the mental health associations and that this was almost exclusively so with regard to the active members. The effective part of the Board, in other words, was a special interest group, self-selected people, each of whom had for one reason or another an interest in mental health and who expressed this by joining a mental health association and so becoming eligible for election.

There were only two members in the entire history of all three Boards who came from blue-collar occupations, and it can be argued that a more vigorous effort ought to have been made to secure a larger representation. Their presence would have been a step closer to the ideal of community in which the "consumer of services determines the kind and nature of mental illness services."[22] It turned out, as might have been predicted from empirical studies by sociologists, that it was exceedingly difficult to get such individuals to join the Board, and those who did were more inclined to be passive spectators than to take an active part.

As it can be seen from Chapter 7, the original plans for the Board called for it to "represent" the population of the area in terms of an arbitrarily designed stratified quota sample. This was in lieu of a random sample that was never seriously considered because it was so obviously impracticable. Selection through a political process of secret ballot and popular election was also bypassed for the same reason. There was not nearly enough interest in mental health or mental illness to make an election possible.

Table 15 makes it evident that the quota sample was not achieved and, hence, that there was no representation in this meaning of the term. The Board might still have "represented" the population in the sense in which a lawyer represents a client. The population of the Centre's geographic area, of course, in no manner employed the Board, but it can be supposed that a board could identify with the people and act as their advocate in matters pertaining to the work of a center. The intent of the Advisory Board, and of those later responsible for the reorganization and reformulation that took place in 1961, was that the Board should be able to present the needs and feelings of the people in the geographic area to the Mental Health Administration and to the staff and that it should also utilize such knowledge in the formulation of its own policies. This was the reason for a membership design that called for participation by elected members of local government and by categories of persons assumed to understand relevant local needs and feelings, namely, physicians and clergy. There was also attention to securing a balanced geographic distribution, at least in terms of the counties served.

It would be wrong to say that this kind of representation did not occur at all, but it is apparent that the Board acted less as an advocate of the client population than as an advocate of the staff. To a degree, it behaved like a barrister, on the basis of information formulated and supplied by the Centre's personnel. Although this is a proper function of a board, up to a point, it is quite different from representing the population and protecting the clients against "the self-serving tendencies of professions."

When one looks at the BB chronologically, it is evident that it went through several phases. The early years from 1961 through 1963 were a period of growth in which the numbers rose from five to twenty members with the loss of only one member. This was also a time when the Board had an exceedingly planful and action-minded chairperson. In 1964, however, he resigned because he had accepted a position in a different part of the country. Immediately after this, there was a period of turnover in which the BB lost eleven members and gained five, resulting in a net loss of six. The situation remained pretty much at this level until approximately 1969, when fourteen members joined and three dropped out.

Through 1970 and 1971 ten new members were added to the BB, and fifteen left. Although some of the departures from the Board were for such reasons as moving to a different area, others appeared to be associated with the emotional tensions between the Board and the staff during the crisis in Bristol described in Chapters 5 and 6. One member, at least, stated explicitly that these tensions were his reason for resigning. It is also noteworthy that of the thirty members who left the BB during the eleven years of our review, half did so at this time. Thus it was that by the end of March 1972, ten of the twenty Board members were newcomers.

As has been pointed out several times, geographic mobility was a factor in depleting and rendering unstable the Board membership. Let us summarize this by saying that of sixty-six area residents who at one point or another joined the Advisory Board, the WG, and the BB, forty-six left the Board, and eighteen of these (39 percent) did so because they left the area. This was, in part, a consequence of the job and career patterns characteristic of small towns. Teachers, engineers, accountants, the managers of local banks and chain stores, and independent businessmen who are striving to get ahead – cosmopolitans, in short – are all apt to move away after a few years of residence. The same, of course, applies to their spouses. Retired cosmopolitans can offset the trend to some extent, but declining energy and failing health place limits on this resource. Thus, although the area served by the Centre was, overall, not one of great population movement, the cosmopolitans who made up an increasing influence on the Board were much at risk in this regard.

Concluding note

The overwhelming evidence, both quantitative and qualitative, is that participation by "the community" in the Board was restricted, unstable and ineffective. As a consequence, the Board did not have the political characteristics necessary for carrying out some of the central requirements of its charge. This situation obtained despite the fact that there was considerable goodwill in the population toward the Centre and its work. Such feelings are attested by the success of the Mental Health Association's annual drives for funds and by the appropriations from town and municipal councils. Many people were apparently willing to give generously but not to become personally involved in long-term commitments and responsibilities. My observations suggest that an important part of this unwillingness was due to that uneasiness about mental illnesses described as barrier two in Chapter 2.

It was also, however, a manifestation of a more general tendency toward low levels of public participation in local governments and voluntary organizations as mentioned earlier in this chapter. There were a number of other groups in Bristol, including the town council, that were having problems very like those of the Board, and there is much to indicate that these problems are widespread in North America. Crises and confrontations call out crowds, but the meetings of boards and councils focused on long-term, regular, often tedious matters necessary for the satisfactory conduct of local affairs go unattended.[23]

Finally, let us observe that in an important sense there was no "community" from which members could be sent to make up the Board. The counties of Harwich, Kingston, and Stirling were each composed of many geographic communities, Stirling alone, as we have seen, having over ninety of them. Among these there was great variation in size, economic resources, occupations, levels of education, culture, sense of being a community, autonomy, and so on and on. Many of the larger ones had distinct feelings of territoriality, so that Board members from one of these areas often struggled against those from another. The effort reported earlier by members from Harwich to move the Centre away from Bristol was one of many such skirmishes. The only way in which the word *community* could be properly used to refer to all the people in the 2,261-square-mile area served at this time by the Centre would be in just one of the meanings given by the Oxford Dictionary: an equivalent of the word *public*. In such a meaning there is little left that approximates in any way the ideal model of a community.

It is noteworthy that in the United States this reality was also forced on the attention of the U.S. National Institute of Mental Health, which fostered many centers. But its implications seem never to have been taken seriously. According to Foley:

Public law 88-164, Section 203, assigned to the NIMH staff the problem of defining the limits of "community." Cain, under Atwell's supervision and with Felix's approval and direction, took on the task. He reviewed the social science literature and contacted several prominent social scientists; neither source agreed on the meaning of the term "community." "We came down to simply 'numbers of people' because the other approaches – political, geographic, ethnic, [sic] or socioeconomic boundaries – did not work. 'Quantities of population' was the last resort."

Foley goes on to describe how NIMH determined what "quantities of population" would mean

Felix had stated in his congressional testimony before Hill and Harris that each center would serve approximately 100,000 persons. He arrived at this figure on the spur of the moment, by simply dividing the two thousand centers discussed in the president's task force into a population of 200,000,000.

Consequently, Cain, Atwell, Brown, and Felix agreed to use that figure as a point of departure, refine the figure, and thus define the parameters of the community in terms of numbers of persons in geographical areas on the basis of economic, clinical, and political criteria. These criteria narrowed the arbitrariness of their definition. From an economic-clinical standpoint, if a community was defined as less than 50,000 persons, the unit costs would be prohibitive; if it was defined as above 200,000 persons, the centers would become mob scenes, and clinicians would be overwhelmed with patients. The political sense of these men dictated that, should they set the minimum figure at 50,000, certain sections of the country would attempt to construct centers "on every corner" and would shortly bankrupt the program. Discussion on the maximum figure ranged from 150,000 persons to 250,000 persons, with little political weight given these figures. In the end, they settled on the range 75,000 to 200,000 persons within given geographical areas.[24]

Thus, the connotations of the largely fictitious ideal community came to be vested in geographic population units of 75,000 to 200,000 people – units that had no necessary community attribute other than occupying a geographic area. It seems that political values and considerations of expediency were so dominant that social scientific information stood little chance of attention. In fact, as Cain says, it was rejected because it "did not work," in other words, did not fit with what the policymakers wanted to do.

We must conclude that the word *community* has a false aura of unified meaning and that it actually refers to a variety of concepts and to numerous exceedingly heterogeneous phenomena. Thus, like *mental health*, it encourages lump thinking and miscommunication. Putting such misleading words together to form *community mental health* could be regarded as amusing were it not for the fact that it has produced much unworkable policy and many shortfalls in care for mentally ill people.

9 The Bristol Centre: the Board and the process of governance

In this chapter we shall examine a number of the factors that affected the governance of the Centre adversely. Emphasis will continue to be on the Board, because the intent of the charge to the Board was to give it a central role and because most of the other subsystems which affected governance interacted with it.

Organization and management within the Board

That there would be problems of organization and management can be seen as inevitable from the quantitative description of the Board given in the previous chapter. The small proportion of active members made it difficult to assemble sufficient numbers of members to transact the Board's business. The requirement for a quorum in the BB and the modal number of active members were the same, namely, seven.

Furthermore, active members were apt to be people who were busy in other organizations as well, a circumstance that placed obstacles in the way of finding meeting times that were feasible for all. There were frequent occasions when the quarterly meetings required in the bylaws – including the annual meeting to elect officers – were not held or were held months after the stipulated date. On one occasion, the Board went for over a year and a half without once getting together. Even when there were regular meetings, the mix of members attending one meeting might be very different from those attending the next. Such discontinuity interfered with developing and maintaining informed and consistent policies. Thus it was that committees were set up to accomplish some task and then forgotten by everyone including the committee chairperson. This may sometimes have been a tactic for avoiding a troublesome decision, but it was also often a matter of inattention. When Board meetings with a quorum present did take place, they tended to focus on accumulated matters that had become urgent, and attention to long-range considerations was repeatedly postponed.

There was considerable variation over time in the effort exerted by Board members to overcome the limits imposed by their small numbers and to achieve efficient organization with attention to agenda preparation, adherence to parliamentary procedures, adequate minute keeping, follow-up on old business, and so forth. There were times when the Board handled these matters well, but on other occasions it was lax in the extreme. This laxity is evident in the incompleteness of many of the Board's transactions. It is also evident that a contributing factor was the dropping out of members without competent replacement.

There was also a factor of chairperson style. Some tried to foster Board growth and the development of its potential. Others acted on their own, ignoring it or manipulating it – much as did some of the Centre directors.

A major handicap to Board functioning was the inclusion of representatives of the Mental Health Administration and the Centre staff as either voting or advisory members. Because of this, the local members never had a Board meeting alone except by accident, and consequently they had almost no opportunity to discuss matters among themselves when formally assembled. This was especially obtrusive when issues of importance were up for consideration, because representatives of the Administration were usually there to listen, and they often intervened before the local Board members had an opportunity to explore each other's ideas and determine their collective thinking. The fact that the director of the Centre was ex officio the secretary meant that he could not only influence what went on at the meetings but could also determine what was entered into the minutes. That the minutes were biased in favor of the staff's viewpoint is demonstrated by editorializing that is now plainly on the record; this bias would have been greater had it not been for occasional demands by Board members for revision and for less biased reporting.

Contributions from Administration and staff were, of course, exceedingly important for the Board's deliberations, but had these individuals appeared only by invitation, the local members could have met by themselves when they chose as a "committee of the whole."

In view of all its organizational difficulties, one might well ask how the Board could function at all. The answer is that it did so through the chairperson or the chairperson plus two or three others acting as an informal, and occasionally formal, executive committee. In this situation, the primary function became that of aiding the director of the Centre in accordance with his requests. It was he, in the main, who determined both short- and long-range policy on the local scene and who did whatever was done to fit the service to local needs. He acquired de facto most of the power and responsibility that, according to the charge, belonged to the Board.

This pattern of functioning made it possible for a Board that was incomplete in numbers and low in attendance to help, nevertheless, in keeping the Centre alive, often doing much more than this in such matters as raising funds and standing up to the Mental Health Administration. By the same token, it was difficult for the Board and its chairperson to turn about and question the staff's policies and actions. The structure of the relationships made it easier for the Board to appease than to control.

Guiding sentiments

The turnover rate in Board membership affected the system of shared sentiments even more than it did matters of organization and management. The sentiments on the whole tended to be diffuse, disconnected, unstable, individual rather than shared, and on some relevant topics nonexistent. It is possible, nonetheless, to make a few generalizations with reference to the original goals and the charge.

By and large, Board members were strongly interested in seeing that something called diagnostic and treatment services were provided to as large a clientele as possible, but they were exceedingly diverse in their grasp of what this meant and in their support of the rest of the goals described in Chapter 4. The concern with diagnosis and treatment was almost certainly due to the fact that the private- and charitable-service models were familiar to virtually all the Board members, whereas the emerging universal-service model was much less so.

The Board's sense of responsibility for providing a service did not extend to the technical and professional aspects of care. The members believed that they had no competence in such matters and, further, that it would be unethical for them to have access to the case records or other personal information about their fellow residents in the area served by the Centre. These matters, they thought, were in the hands of the professional staff, whereas questions of staff competence and the maintenance of standards rested with the Mental Health Administration.

The goals of referral, consultation, outreach, and development of area resources were thought by the Board to be closely related to the provision of services, but the members also thought that for the most part decisions in these matters should be made by the staff. The Board was very willing to accept staff suggestions and back them up as formally adopted policy.

Prevention and research, although enthusiastically supported by some Board members, were viewed with uncertainty or skepticism by others.[1] Training and university ties were seen as important by very few of the members, although many were favorably disposed toward the Stirling

County Study and thought that this particular university link brought a number of practical benefits to the Centre and to the area. Some of the Board members felt they did not understand what the Study "was really doing," and this increased with time as those members who had been part of the Centre's founding were replaced by others, some of whom were not only little aware of the originating experiences and ideas but were also newcomers to the area.

William Mayer-Gross, the outstanding German psychiatrist and exile from Nazi Germany, has left a vivid record of his impressions and aims during his time at the Crichton Royal Hospital in Dumfriesshire, Scotland. As described by Aubrey Lewis, the spirit of this institution had some resemblance to that of the Bristol Mental Health Centre. He refers to it as "easy-going" and "bucolic" and as being "neither the seat nor affiliate of a university." In striving for excellence, Mayer-Gross was troubled by the absence of "full clinical observation," "documentation in well-kept case records," and "clinical research into the course and causation of diseases." In particular, he deplored the lack of

academic vivacity, conviviality and competition which is to be found even in the smallest university or school of medicine as a natural by-product of the gathering of young minds. Thus it would be difficult for me to calculate the amount of time and effort I spent for the sole purpose of attracting the right people as collaborators in research; to rouse and keep the interest of young psychiatrists in the work they had taken up; and to fill by adequate replacement the gaps left by those who tended away from their loneliness of country life.[2]

Very few of the Board members in Bristol after the formation of the BB in 1961 had any inkling of the kind of thing Mayer-Gross was talking about or its pertinence to good patient care. Similarly, despite continuing informational efforts by the Stirling County Study, there were few Board members who were aware of the points presented by the Centre director in 1956 to the Mental Health Administration, as reported in Chapter 7 and Appendix B.

Some of the reasons lay in the difficulty the personnel of the Stirling County Study had keeping fully acquainted with the changing Board members, in the Board's problem of finding times to meet, in the Administration's increasingly negative attitude toward the presence of the Stirling County Study after 1961, and in the gradual recruitment of a staff that was largely antiacademic. The influence of the Stirling County Study was still further weakened in 1970 when it tried to dissuade the staff from participating in the school issue. After that, the Study was treated more or less openly as an enemy by the staff and as "controversial" by some Board members. The Board was also, of course, affected by the local and

national tide of antiintellectual, antiprofessional, and antielitist sentiments described in Chapter 5.

Although the Board members believed that mental health work was a
good thing and that their mission was to keep the Centre alive, mental
illness was clearly a topic that made them uneasy. The various mental
illness syndromes were rarely mentioned at meetings, and then only in the
most general terms. The members were not eager to hear about the differential numbers of the disorders in the population, the modes of treatment,
or research into causes, courses and outcomes. The words *mental health*
provided a way to avoid frank and explicit discussion of mental illnesses
and the problems they posed for individuals and for the society of the
area. The members appeared to want to help reduce or stamp out mental
illnesses but to do so while talking about them as little as possible. Although it is very likely that thinking about any malignant and threatening
disease makes most people uneasy, it is hard to imagine a hospital board
that would to the same extent use *health* when it actually meant flu epi-
demics, heart disease, strokes and cancer.

The disadvantages of euphemistic and optimistic terms in the deliberations of bodies such as the Board were well stated as long ago as 1952 by
Buell:

Our own use of pathological terminology is deliberate, however, because we believe it is conducive to more precise thinking. Pathological conditions exist, it is
possible to get data about them, study their causation, observe and test efforts to
correct them and prevent their occurrence. The practical danger of using more
optimistic sounding phrases lies not only in the fact that the concepts may be more
vague, but also, and more importantly, in the fact that a program which does not
accept ultimate responsibility for the prevention or protection against pathology
conditions is removed from the compulsion to measure specific results.[3]

The Centre's Board, because it followed the common terminology of
the mental health movement, was inhibited in achieving anything more
than a very imprecise understanding of what the staff it directed either
was doing or should be doing. The staff, for its part, encouraged this as a
defense against interference by the Board.

Substantive knowledge

Most Board members most of the time had very little factual knowledge
about the mental health and mental illness field. In evaluating this lack,
one has to be mindful of the field's enormous extent, ill-defined boundaries, and increasingly conflictful content. To be really on top of the subject matter and live up to the responsibilities of the charge would have

meant something like a half-time commitment by each Board member – which is, to say the least, expecting a great deal from volunteers. As Kaplan has said:

Citizen participation, as the meaningful involvement of individuals in significant organizational events, is not readily achieved. In our modern society, participation means a personal commitment of time and effort without guarantees of security. It requires training for ill defined functions by an educational process not geared to the task. It also requires an involvement in organizational relationships dependent upon traditions no longer as binding as they were and for which a new ethic has yet to evolve.[4]

In stating that the Board did not do well in acquiring or utilizing substantive knowledge, it is also important to note that there were at all times individuals who were highly informed and who worked hard to keep themselves up to date. Despite this, however, lack of knowledge in the Board as a whole contributed heavily to dependence on the staff for information, interpretation, and decision, and to the fact that when knowledgeable individual Board members put forward recommendations that were opposed by the staff, the majority of the Board as a rule disregarded them and went along with the staff. The dead weight of ignorance was formidable.

One of the major deficiencies in Board knowledge was its poor grasp of the seriousness of the Centre's work. They thought of the Centre as a place where those who felt depressed and anxious could be helped and where troublesome psychological quirks could be straightened out. A few people no doubt looked upon the Centre's work as trivial because they believed it to consist of pampering complainers whose main problem was lack of "guts" and who "by rights" ought to "snap out of it" on their own. In the main, however, the Board members pictured the Centre as engaged in a very worthy type of help giving but one that did not involve risk to life. They thought of staff activity as helpful or as failing to help but not really as ever able to do much harm.

In actual fact, the Centre did deal with a small but steady volume of illnesses and situations in which a wrong decision could be and sometimes was fatal. As illustrated in Table 1 (see Chapter 4), about a quarter of the admissions to the Centre were psychotic. Among these, a small but significant number were extremely suicidal. A smaller but still significant number were homicidal, and a larger number were at risk for incurring or causing fatal accidents. In cases of this kind, the survival of the patient and of others may well hang on skill in diagnosis and adequacy of case management in terms of such matters as psychotherapy, medication, electroshock, hospitalization, and advice to family members and the family physician. What is required is the control of the consequences of delusions, hallucinations, inner preoccupations at the expense of outer awareness, and surges of overwhelming emotions such as rage, grief, and elation. There was, for example, in Stirling County during the period of our study a student who, apparently in a state of exultation, climbed a pole and burned his arms off to the elbows by grabbing high-tension wires; a woman who tried several times to kill her husband because of a delusion that he intended to kill their child; a taxi driver who while driving was subject to sudden episodes of disorientation and blind rage; and a man with a long history of psychotic preoccupation with religious delusions who was accidentally killed on the highway by a car – most likely in a spell of preoccupation.[5] Less direct but nonetheless vital were numerous problems of survival for children in families in which a parent was psychotic or severely retarded.

Again as indicated by Table 1 (Chapter 4), nearly half of the patients admitted to the Centre suffered from psychoneuroses. The great bulk of these involved symptoms of anxiety, fatigue, nervousness, and depression and would be classified as mild affective disorders according to DSM III. From time to time, however, there were a few who, though not psychotic in their symptomatology, were nevertheless suicidal risks and in need of penetrating understanding and careful case management.

Aside from the life-threatening attributes of the mental illnesses themselves, the ability of the clinician to make a differential diagnosis was on occasion a matter upon which life and death could depend. Thus, some organic disorders can first appear as complaints and behaviors that are very like depression and anxiety. Brain tumors, for instance, have now and then been mistaken for depression until long after the time during which surgical intervention could have been successful. The general practitioners in Stirling County not infrequently sought help from the Centre staff in making this kind of discrimination.

Securing compliance to a treatment regime from a patient and his or her family is another area in which the ability of the clinician can make a difference not only to health but also to life, at least in the more severe types of illnesses. From the mid-1950s onward, the development of medications has greatly increased the clinician's ability to bring about improvements in mental illnesses. But there are concomitant new dangers as well, as mentioned in Chapter 5. Misapplication and failure to monitor by a clinician can result in crippling damage to the brain and other organs and to death.

The Board's lack of concern about these risks to life that were inherent in the activities of the Centre staff was again due in part to the first barrier described in Chapter 2 – namely, unawareness of the heterogeneity of the field covered by the term mental health. In consequence, the milder and more positive connotations of the phrase obscured the fact that it also referred to life-threatening disorders that called for high levels of skill if grave errors were to be avoided. Our case study supports the view that the present-day emphasis among mental health workers on "problems of living" and the notion that mental illnesses are not real can and does lead to neglecting serious mental illnesses with injurious, sometimes disastrous consequences.

The Board's difficulties in acquiring and utilizing information, of course, had many causes. A number of these were outlined in the discussion in the two preceding chapters about the Board's origin, history, numerical weakness, and structural instability. To these factors may now be added the fact that the members were in no way screened and selected for ability to delve, to sift, and to reach balanced decisions. Nor was any guidance available to them as to how to go about solving the kinds of issues that confronted them. No one played a role analogous to that of a judge instructing a jury about the handling of evidence and the objectives to bear in mind. Systematic efforts to inform new Board members regarding what they needed to know were not provided by the Stirling County Study, the provincial Mental Health Association, or the provincial Mental Health Administration. Although the public health officers of the relevant areas (as representatives of the Administration) sat on the Board, their lack of training in psychiatry made it impossible for them to be of very much help. They were also muted by the common reluctance of civil servants to speak out on any topic that could prove controversial and so have political repercussions that might be harmful to them. Thus, all in all, the Board was not well selected, well informed, or well advised.

For a time during the early sixties, one of the long-standing members, who had been on the original Advisory Board, and the Centre director made some effort to inform new Board members, but the communications were entirely verbal. No brochure was prepared, nor any file of annual reports, and there was never a committee with responsibility for meeting and leading discussions with new members. For several years the Board member mentioned above also conducted annual seminars designed to help people update their knowledge in fields broadly related to the problems of mental health, but these were very little attended by other members. This experience, together with the chronic difficulty the Board had in assembling for its regular meetings, prompts the impression that even had informative sessions been provided, it is unlikely that they would have been much attended.

The concept of boards composed of local citizens controlling services does not include the demand that the members of such boards become experts in technical and professional knowledge. It does, however, include the idea that the members will strive to understand the basic principles involved in the issues they face, will gather all the relevant information available, and will utilize, when appropriate, a variety of expert opinions. Their deliberating together according to formal procedures is expected to mitigate personal biases and impulsive leaping to conclusions.

The ability of the Centre's Board to perform in this manner varied at different times, mostly depending on the chairperson. Under some chairpersons issues were studied, tough questions were asked, and knowledgeable people were consulted. At least these things were done by the chairperson and a few colleagues; the rest of the Board did little more than look on. Under other chairpersons, there was a heavy reliance not only on the staff but also on preset opinions that were triggered by surface aspects of the issues. Most notable was a tendency to personalize – that is, to see differences in points of view as personality clashes and, in extreme instances, to categorize the proponents as good people and bad people. The deliberations were often essentially social and emotional transactions among the Board and staff members present, sometimes leaning toward achieving a consensus as quickly as possible and sometimes toward allowing recognition-seeking displays by one or another individual. It often seemed that the primary task of patient care was in actuality secondary to caring for the feelings and wishes of Board and staff members.

Close personal acquaintance with a mental illness was also a factor that disturbed the Board's ability to utilize substantive knowledge. One of the reasons people become interested in mental health is the experience of having a mentally ill person in the family or of having been a patient oneself, and such experiences characterized a sprinkling of the Board members. For some, this meant a psychological investment in seeing the staff's activities in a favorable light and an inclination to think in terms of personal loyalty first and foremost. A few had distinctly hostile feelings as a result of their experiences with mental illness care, and one at least thought the Board should fire a certain member of the staff; but, for the most part, such negatively oriented people avoided being members of the Board. The main effect of emotional tension between Board and staff over issues about patient care was to create extreme discomfort among those who had close personal associations with mental illnesses and to induce them to stay away from the Board meetings, and in some cases to resign.

For other Board members, there were additional psychological reasons for reluctance to ask questions when the Centre did not seem to be running as well as it should. These pertained to two of the mental health special-interest group's main goals: educational effort to gain public recognition for the importance of mental health work, and striving for greater development of mental health services. These orientations rendered some Board members exceedingly unwilling to probe. It would be unfair to say that they advocated "covering up" problems but not, perhaps, to say that they thought it better not to know some things.

At the risk of repeating a point that has already been made several times, it is important to emphasize that my description and analysis is not intended to lay blame on individuals. The aim is, rather, to identify and illuminate generic problems of social and psychological processes that must be taken into account if policymaking and planning for the care of mental illnesses are to be improved. An example of such a problem is the topic before us, namely, the frequent inability of boards of directors to muster the information necessary for sound decision making, or even for realizing that there is a decision that ought to be made. That the boards of institutions charged with caring for mental illnesses have had this problem for a long time is suggested by the picturesque words of Weir Mitchell written almost a hundred years ago:

The psychology of boards is as yet unstudied. It is not in the textbooks. The best of them get wooden . . . All boards age rapidly and acquire young the senile characterics. They assimilate with difficulty and abhor change . . . Yet no one thinks these honest gentlemen either stupid or undutiful. They merely do not know their business and do not know that they do not know.[6]

In our own day, Klein and Lewis have noted in their study of community health councils in Britain the discrepancy between the demands of the task and the knowledge, skills, and time available to the individual council members. As a consequence of this (and other related factors), the councils are seen as failing to function adequately:

It is often assumed that locally-controlled services can be equated with accessible, responsive and open services: what might be called a democratic style of administration. But while there may be strong arguments in favour of decentralization – particularly on the grounds that government is now overloaded – it cannot be taken for granted that the result would be to encourage these particular values. The little evidence that is available points in the opposite direction: it suggests that local authorities are perceived to be less responsive and less open than central government.[7]

It is important not to be, or even to seem to be, hard on well-meaning people, lest necessary motivations be damaged. It is equally important, however, for well-meaning people to realize that good intentions are not enough. Knowing what and knowing how are also essential.

Nor should the outside observer be satisfied with either condemning or forgiving individuals such as board members. Both actions are irrelevant because they are dead ends insofar as bringing about improvement is concerned. The intent of the behavioral-science approach of this book is to understand why things go wrong in order to find ways and means for making them go better. The Board of the Bristol Mental Health Centre was an organization set up to accomplish goals that involved the care of numerous individuals and the survival of a few. It fell short for multiple reasons, some of which were inherent in the structure and functioning of the organization itself. The hope is that wider understanding of the processes involved will lead to the more effective functioning of similar organizations in the future through modification of the goals, or through more realistic planning, or both.

Influences external to the Board

The multiple factors just discussed, mainly inherent in the Board itself, placed many obstacles in the Board's way. These were more than matched by a host of external influences which, drawing on Chapter 2, may be summarized as lack of consensus as to what is to be considered mental illness, diverse views regarding treatment, insufficient manpower, underestimation of task magnitude, disrupting waves of interest in fashionable magical solutions, professional claims of omniscience, and both individual and institutional tendencies toward the Lord Ronald syndrome.

The Board came into existence at a point in history when the problem of consensus in the mental health field was becoming rapidly more severe. A review of the literature from 1967 to 1969 by Gottesfeld produced the following illustrative statements:[8]

A community mental health center should treat everyone, regardless of their age, psychiatric diagnosis or degree of disturbance.

Mass treatment or mass prevention methods in psychiatry will only lead to disappointments.

Community mental health programs are committed to political positions rather than health concerns.

A community mental health center should be hospital-centered.

The establishment of community mental health centers will result in ordinary problems of living being interpreted as psychiatric problems.

Concomitant with a kaleidoscopic increase of mostly incompatible convictions about mental health and mental illness, there was also the shift in Canadian society from the private- and charitable-service models of health care toward the universal-service model, with results that were a hodgepodge of all three models (see Chapter 5).

Under the wide arch of such conflicting views and ideologies, there were a number of more local conditions that also interfered with the Board's ability to define its objectives and develop consistent patterns of action. Thus, the Mental Health Administration produced no memorandum of understanding in which was stated the relationships between itself and the Board. This absence helped to foster a feeling in the Board of never knowing where it stood with the Administration or how to interpret the latter's pronouncements. Rightly or wrongly, the Board perceived the Administration as inclined to change the meaning of its words while maintaining that it had not done so but that the Board had "misunderstood." Sleight-of-hand with words is easy and tempting when the terms employed are mental illness, mental health, community, and prevention.

Before making a judgment about the Administration, however, it is well to realize that it, too, was subject to all the major problems just listed. In addition, it had the task of surviving as a social subsystem by staying on top of the quicksilver surface of political processes. Nor should we lose sight of the administrator's dedication to the development of mental health services despite the fact that the topic never had very strong political appeal – the hard work of the mental health associations notwithstanding. My aim here, as with the Board, is not to blame or praise but rather to point out patterns of behavior that, whatever their origins and justifications, had numbing consequences. Even had the Board had no intrinsic malfunctions, these multiple extrinsic problems would likely have been sufficient to cripple it.

A second negative influence was one for which I shall borrow the term *double bind* from a well-known theory about the cause of schizophrenia.[9] The theory holds that it is psychologically destructive for an individual to receive from a person powerful in his life demands that are mutually incompatible, that is, that put him in a "can't win" predicament.

The words and actions of the Mental Health Administration did just this to the Board. For example, the administrator was quoted in the minutes of the inaugural meeting of the BB as saying that the Board was to be "self-governing, having the power to make its own policies, and set out its own programmes, a responsible body fit to receive and account for public monies." The Board was also called a "corporate authority with powers to make decisions." These views were repeated at subsequent meetings. The Board, however, discovered that when it tried to behave in this self-governing manner and did things not in accord with the Administration's wishes, a threat that funds would be withheld was made. Thus, even though it meant amending its already legally established *Memorandum of Association*, the Board felt forced to rescind its edict that the administrator and the public health officers were advisory members only and to reinstate them as full voting members. Numerous decisions involving such matters as travel money, the purchase of books and equipment for the Centre, and staff leave met with objections from the Administration and were subject at times to reversal. On such occasions, instead of speaking of the Board's "authority and power to make decisions," the Administration pointed to the amount of money it was supplying and to its responsibility to see "how it was spent, and why."

These financial discussions with the administrator during board meetings were sometimes reported in the minutes as "heated." It is apparent that the Administration's pattern of pointing to Board authority and at the same time exerting control through the purse strings was a source of continuing discontent and bewilderment to the Board and took up time that could have been spent more constructively.

An episode occurred in 1961 that a number of Board members believed exposed the real viewpoint of the provincial government lurking beneath its statements about Board authority. According to the minutes of a meeting held on November 4th, a letter came from the provincial government's health grant office stipulating that if the Board wished to receive its money it must in the future inform the head of that office when meetings were to be held. The most interesting thing was that the letter did not use the word *board*, but substituted for it the phrase *advisory committee*. The chairman replied by pointing out that the Board was a legally constituted body and not an advisory committee and, further, that the head of the health grants office was not a member and therefore was not eligible for notification of when meetings were to be held. No more was heard from the grants office, but the episode did not improve relations between the Board and the Administration or help the Board to achieve a clearer definition of itself and its task.

There were other ways besides the purse strings through which the Administration undermined the Board. For example, it was clearly understood that the director of the Centre was an employee of the Board and was responsible to it. Yet members of the Administration frequently met with the staff in the absence of Board representatives, made decisions, and told the Board about them afterward. Or again, the Administration said that one of the Board's functions was to shape activities of the Centre so they would meet the particular needs of, and rise to the particular opportunities in, its geographic area. Indeed, this was pointed up as a major reason for having a Board. Yet, when the Board attempted to do this, it was told that all the centers in the province had to operate according to the same pattern and that there could be no special features.

In 1961, the Administration for the first time produced a draft of its manual of *Policies and Regulations with Regard to Grants-in-Aid to Community Mental Health Boards.* Despite the fact that the document was called a draft, the Board felt it was a unilateral statement and was much annoyed. The members believed that if a board had the responsibility the Administration said it had, then it must have a say in the promulgation of the rules and criteria for decision making. Instead of that, they had been handed a detailed document that, the Board claimed, the Administration was not ready to alter in any fundamental way.

This feeling on the part of the Board was not, perhaps, altogether justified, for the Administration did revise the manual to some extent, and the finished statement was not issued until the following year. The Board, however, remained unsatisifed, saying that the manual was cast in such general terms as to give the Administration leeway with interpretation that still left the Board without a firm understanding of what it could and could not do. The manual failed, in the Board's opinion, to remedy the basic situation by which the members were given responsbility without authority. They said the Administration was trying to use them as a "rubber stamp" for its policies. This could be put a different way by saying that, being very short of staff, the Administration was trying to use the Board as a device for achieving certain features of local management at low cost while retaining power in its own hands.

That this, rather than representation, was in the thinking of the Administration is more than hinted in its own description of board organization and structure:

The management of each Centre is in the hands of a local Board of responsible citizens who accept its administrative, financial and legal responsibilities . . . [T]hey are not psychiatric professionals. Our feeling is that a community mental health project, to function as it should, must have lay members in control. *If properly chosen,* they are in a much better *position to "influence the community."*[10] (italics added)

Plainly, the direction of influence in mind was from the Administration downward and not upward from the community.

The double bind had the effect of lowering morale, discouraging participation, and watering down the Board's control of the staff. It also had the effect of uniting Board and staff in a struggle against the vagaries of what they perceived to be a common enemy. In this battle, the Centre director tended to be the strategist and to play a dominant role, even though the negotiations were formally conducted by the Board.

Again in fairness to the Administration, one must note that there were enough weaknesses in the Board to justify apprehension and cause changes of mind. At the same time, it is well to remember that the double bind was, through its demoralizing effect, a significant contributor to many of those Board weaknesses that gave the Administration pause.

The situation in which only a small number of individuals out of the total population of the area served by the Centre were willing to be members of the Board is probably not a rare occurrence. Such is indicated by the American Psychiatric Association's statement that "In many communities there has been little or no community participation in developing the center or determining what services are needed." On the other hand, those who did participate in boards often found it frustrating and would likely have endorsed the further comment of the Association that "lack of opportunities for the ordinary citizen to take part in policy-making had helped encourage public apathy and distrust of government and other programming."[11]

At the Bristol Centre, these two trends appeared to reinforce each other: public "apathy" or minimal interest encouraged administrators to exert control lest the enterprise collapse, and "bureaucratic" behavior dampened the never very strong interest of the public. In fairness to both Administration and Board, the reader may be reminded once more, as discussed in Chapter 5, of the sea of increasing uncertainty in which together they were exploring and seeking task definition and effective administrative organization.

The double bind has been given emphasis here not only because of its malfunctional consequences in the operation of the Centre but also because it is a mischief-making process that has wide distribution. I have, for example, observed it in the administration of the Bureau of Indian Affairs in the United States. Here, too, the announced policy was the formation of autonomous bodies (tribal councils) and the turning of authority over to them so that "the people could be self-governing." Administrative tactics, however, involved retention of control through the manipulation of purse strings and the use of ambiguous statements in order to maintain room for maneuvering. The result was a double bind that infuriated the Indians and laid a dead hand on self-government. When it came to power, it was the government that was the "Indian giver."

The medical subsystem of the geographic area served by the Centre contributed to the Board's problems, as we have seen, by turning away from the part originally expected of it. The medical associations in both

Harwich and Kingston Counties refused to nominate members to the Board. In Stirling County, although a physician played a leading role in the formation of the Board, following reorganization in 1961 physicians ceased to participate.

The doctors did, however, communicate often and freely with the director of the Centre for a time, until the troubles of the later years developed and separation began. Discussions were mostly about particular patients, but the doctors also expressed views and preferences from time to time about matters they thought the Centre should or should not take into account. Consequently, such advice and guidance as the Board received from the doctors of the area was through the Centre's director.

There were two main reasons that the physicians did not wish to sit on the Centre's Board. One was a disinclination to become involved in anything that looked like expanding government influence in medical affairs; the other was a related desire not to join with laymen in making policy decisions that could affect other doctors, in this case the psychiatrists in the Centre. The feeling that dictated these decisions had been growing as part of the struggle over the advance toward universal medical service. Thus, although the medical staff of the local general hospital had for many years had a representative on the hospital board, in the early sixties the doctors withdrew from this participation.

For the Board, this meant deprivation of local medical guidance and left it almost wholly dependent on its staff in such matters. The medical attitudes expressed by silence and absence, furthermore, did nothing to enhance the Board's self-esteem, but rather encouraged it to lean over backward to avoid trespassing in forbidden medical pathways. At the same time, it annoyed a good many of the Board members and bred some resentment among them toward the doctors together with a feeling of "We'll get along better without them." This prepared the way for siding with the Centre staff when the doctors became concerned about patient care at the Centre.

The Stirling County Study, during the first years of the Board's existence, endeavored to supply it with whatever information, advice, and practical aid appeared appropriate. By degrees, however, the Study diminished its participation in the administrative affairs of the Centre, based on the theory that the Board would better and more quickly learn its role and functions if it were not dependent on the Study. The Board felt the same way and, hence, it was mutually agreeable in the reorganization of 1961 for the representative of the Study to become an advisory rather than a voting member.

A consequence of this, however, was that from this time onward the

Study's contacts were primarily with the staff. The intent was to avoid any semblance of going over the staff's head to the Board. Thus, in essence, the Study became an advisory group not to the Board but to the staff. Through most of this period (up to the time of the school issue), it was the director of the Centre who controlled the flow of information and suggestions from the Study to the Board.

At the beginning in 1956, the staff, like the Stirling County Study, had been idealistic in its view of the Board and had worked hard to help it become a successful example of local leadership in the mental illness field. With time and staff turnover, however, these feelings changed. The actions of the Mental Health Administration and the doctors of the area were not, of course, lost on the staff, and this, together with observing Board weaknesses, encouraged a feeling that the Board should be pro forma, with the director of the Centre constituting the real decision maker. Both the staff and the Administration, in short, competed in efforts to use the Board as a rubber stamp for their separate and often conflicting aims.

Staff pro forma treatment of the Board is illustrated by an occasion on which the director hired and then fired an individual many months before submitting either transaction to the Board. This meant that the Board was asked to approve first the hiring and then the firing of the same individual at the same meeting. On a number of occasions, the Board made important requests of the staff that were ignored. Examples were proposals for homemaker services and for organizing the parents of retarded children. It was not a matter of the staff advising against these proposals for such and such reasons. There was simply no response at all.

The attitude of the staff can be summed up by saying that, like virtually all such social units, it worked toward its own autonomy, employing the Board at times as a shield and at times as a sword in its dealings with the Administration, but otherwise acting as if the Board had no authority.

The local mental health associations were highly important to the Centre, but it is necessary to say little more about them from the point of view of Centre functioning. This is because, as indicated in the previous chapter, active Board members and leaders in the mental health associations were for the most part the same individuals. What has been said about the strengths and weaknesses of the Board, therefore, was also essentially true of the associations.

The legal subsystem had little if any direct influence. In the realm of climate of opinion, however, it had an indirect effect that touched many aspects of the Centre's working. During the sixties, there was a growth of legal sentiment that looked sharply at anything that might be construed as unfair treatment of an employee. This went so far as to raise questions in general hospitals about the power of senior physicians to discipline younger physicians for inadequate care of patients. The Ontario Royal Commission's Inquiry into Civil Rights referred to such disciplinary actions as "private professional penal justice" and suggested that it "should be withdrawn and all disciplinary matters decided by the courts of law."[12]

In harmony with this legal viewpoint was a value in the counterculture movement that opposed strongly any act that could be defined as depriving a person of the "right to self-respect." Such opinions were given pointed local meaning because of a bitter attack being conducted some fifty miles from Bristol by a physician against a hospital board that had withdrawn his hospital privileges. This hospital's decision prevailed, but at a cost of great discomfort to the Board and to the medical staff that supported the Board.

Concluding note

It is apparent that the Board paralleled the staff in relinquishing most of the original goals and concentrating on a rather traditional pattern of service: a free, basically charitable clinic that offered help to troubled people. In the course of this relinquishment of original goals, it largely overlooked serious mental illnesses.

Although the Board with its charge began in the vanguard of those wishing to provide universal service for a geographic area, it grew conservative in this respect as its membership and the membership of the staff changed and it fell behind national trends. Its main attention became focused on budgetary matters and on negotiations with the Mental Health Administration about working conditions for the staff rather than on patient care, outreach, and so forth. Long-range planning and policymaking were displaced by immediate concerns. The orientation was one that set the highest priority on keeping the Centre in existence. Virtually the entire sense of mission became concentrated on this point. As a consequence, all other aspects of the Board's charge suffered. Notably, it ignored questions of competence, and, although called a Board of Directors, it failed to direct. In this it behaved in many ways like the consumer-based boards of health centers described by Paap. These, too, were dominated and largely neutralized by professionals and other related translocal networks of influence.[13]

Additional reasons for this state of affairs can be grouped under the word *manpower*, if this is understood to include relevant capabilities as well as numbers of bodies. Analysis of the quantitative data demonstrates that the Board suffered from insufficient numbers and from turnover in membership, with derivative problems of basic knowledge, organization, and management. When the manpower problems of the Board are seen in relation to those of the staff and of the Mental Health Administration, it is apparent that from top to bottom the province's mental health enterprise suffered from chronic numerical weakness. It never had the personnel necessary for the fulfilling of its goals and the implementation of its plans.

In discussing the Centre as a foreign body in the community's social system in Chapter 7, I pointed to three categories of sentiments that existed in the population: positive, indifferent, and negative. One of our hopes in establishing a Board was that conversion of the Centre from a foreign body to an integral part of the social system would increase positive attitudes and greatly reduce the other two categories. Later events showed that the Board did help make the Centre more a part of the social system than it had been but that a major reduction of indifference in the population did not follow. Being part of the area's social system meant that the Centre became imbued with the characteristics of that system. These included some of the malfunctioning of social organization that has been described and a lack of strong shared sentiments about mental health and mental illnesses.

In other words, if one succeeds in making a new organization a genuine part of a local social system, one should be prepared to see the organization acquire the negative as well as the positive attributes of that particular system. Both the Board and the social system in which it was set, and from which its members came, suffered from the hindrances to and malfunctions in self-management that have been outlined in the previous chapter in the discussion of the community concept.

10 The behavior of social systems

It was remarked at the beginning of Chapter 5 that the story of the Bristol Mental Health Centre was influenced by vast social forces. Some of these were then illustrated in the accounts of the mental health movement, the trends in the medical profession, and the unrest in and social disintegration of populations in the 1960s (with the crisis over the school issue as an exemplar). The discussion of communities in Chapter 8 also dealt with social forces that had an impact on the functioning of the Centre. In the present chapter, I shall focus attention on some of the patterns common in care-giving agencies and small groups such as boards and committees and touch on relevant aspects of individual motivation.

All these various processes, from mental health movement to agency behavior, are interrelated and are set in the still wider frame of society at large, which can also be understood as having coherence and meaning. I shall begin the chapter, therefore, with a brief panoramic overview of society as a whole and then take up care-giving agencies and small groups. At the end, against the background of these observations, I shall review and analyze the deadlock in which the Bristol Mental Health Centre found itself in the early 1970s.

Society at large

The outstanding feature of modern society is its *rapid rate of change*. The mainsprings of social change probably lie in the interplay of technological innovation, population increase, and accumulating scientific knowledge. Some of the consequences are beneficial to humanity, whereas others range from hazardous to lethal. Increased leisure and life expectancy, smaller families, more women in the work force, mood-altering drugs, birth control pills, organ transplants, industrial automation, exhaustion of energy sources, pollution, and the threat of nuclear war – these phenomena illustrate the developments that shape life today. Particularly relevant to our purposes is the phenomenon of geographic mobility; large numbers

176

of individuals moving from place to place in pursuit of opportunity or keeping their families in one locality and working in another. Cities throughout the world have become overcrowded, and now many rural areas are being filled by a reverse trend.[1]

Meanwhile, the streams of new knowledge and new ideas that have accompanied these changes call into question traditional beliefs and practices across the board, from child rearing to religion. The new knowledge, in turn, becomes obsolete under successive waves of additional discoveries, and the new ideas are themselves displaced by waves of change in fashions of thinking and believing.

Human societies have a remarkable capacity for adapting to innovations and altered circumstances. The speed at which they can do so, however, is limited. It takes time for individuals to assimilate new ways and still longer for them to become socially coordinated. At base, the process is doubtless tied to the biologically fixed response and learning rates of the central nervous system. When social changes are swiftly piled one upon another, therefore, the adaptive capacities of individuals, and hence of society, are exceeded, and social disintegration results. Social processes become fragmented, and things do not work well in the economic, political, or human services spheres. From the point of view of the individual, jobs appear insecure, other people unpredictable, and the institutions of society undependable, be they in health, education, welfare, commerce, or industry.

These changes in the structure of society at large are accompanied by alterations in the sentiments – that is, the systems of belief and values – by which people set their goals, guide their lives, and distinguish between right and wrong. One can see these alterations in the weakening of many traditional religions, the swarming of transient, mystical cults, and the return to fundamentalist religion.

Sentiment change extends into secular realms as well, so that individuals grow conflicted about ethical principles and unsure of standards. The effects are felt in the professions, the courts, corporations, small businesses, and government. There is a tendency for moral behavior to drop below the level of previous norms and for unethical practices to become accepted because "everyone does it." After all, who knows what constitutes allowable behavior in a society in which all conventions appear to be in flux? When is it proper to intervene and attempt control and when is such action an invasion of individual rights? Included in the puzzling over allowable behavior is renewed uncertainty about what is and is not insanity.

Uncertainty breeds apprehension. The more an individual is surrounded by people and events that are perceived to be unpredictable, undependable, and incomprehensible, the more that individual is apt to feel powerless and threatened. These reactions are soon followed by apathy and hopelessness or anger and resentment. In the latter states of mind, people search for scapegoats, fall easily into patterns of suspiciousness and hostility to other groups, and readily seek expression through nationalism, separatism, radicalism, cults, and crises.

At this point it is advisable to qualify. We should remind ourselves that, according to the evidence of history, the management of human affairs has rarely if ever been shiningly efficient. One of the great problems has always been tension between personal inclinations and the duties to others that are inherent in group living. An effective balance between individual rights and individual obligations is hard to achieve and easily lost. Aristotle tells in his *Ethics* that he analyzed the constitutions of 159 Greek city-states without, apparently, finding one that was satisfactory.

Ever since some point in evolution when man, like the wolf, began to run in packs (probably in order to deal better with large prey and enemies), individual survival and individual opportunity have depended on maintaining a place in a social group of some kind. The creation of systematic ways of dividing and coordinating the tasks of group living and the welding of them into societies and cultures has enabled human beings to go beyond attack and defense to more sweeping environmental conquest and to the development of philosophy, religion, the arts, science, and humanism. Great visions of what might be achieved by collective effort have thus come into being.

But the base is an uneasy one. The psychological makeup of man is in many ways ill-fitted to the harness of living in sociocultural systems. Robert B. Edgerton, writing as an anthropologist, puts the matter thus: "Man has a nature which is not entirely tractable and which continues to assert itself no matter what form his culture may take. One aspect of his nature is willfulness, and a concern with self-interest that leads, when conditions are right, to deviance."[2] In striving to satisfy their individual inclinations, people default, cheat, and pillage one another with results that recurrently mar the functioning of societies and cultures and that subvert their institutions and programs. People also give of themselves altruistically and faithfully, and this giving helps to slow down or neutralize the destructive tendencies. On the whole, therefore, societies have, through the ages, hobbled unevenly along, sometimes distinguishing and sometimes extinguishing themselves.

Thus, the state of society today should not be seen as a contrast to some previous ideal state. On the contrary, the problems of today are age-old difficulties greatly enhanced by new sets of social conundrums. Even the rapid rate of change and its attendant consequences has some historical depth, for it has been noted with misgiving by innumerable writers since the eighteenth century. John Hawkes, for instance, writing in 1857 said the following:

I doubt if ever the history of the world . . . could show a larger amount of insanity than that of the present day. It seems, indeed, as if the world was moving at an advanced rate of speed proportionate to its approaching end; as though, in this rapid race of time, increasing with each revolving century, a higher pressure is engendered in the minds of men.[3]

Care-giving agencies

One of the surprising aspects of human organizations is their ability to disregard the goals that are the reason for their existence.[4] Over and over again they make of secondary or less importance the ends to which they are supposedly dedicated and, instead, become immersed in tangential concerns. Thus, many details of running a school system become more important than teaching children; procedures in a court become more important than justice; prestige and hierarchy in a church become more important than Christian conduct; organization in a hospital becomes more important than the care of patients; and administration of an agency becomes more important than delivering to people quality service. Even in the military, despite all the power invested in its authoritarian hierarchy, there is always a difference between what is commanded and what is actually done – a reality made up of concession, accommodation, compromise, and the deliberate ignoring of error.

This property of human organizations is manifest across a wide range of services from agricultural extension to hospitals and clinics. It occurs because all such institutions are subsystems of society at large, each struggling for survival and maintenance of identity while being intermeshed with other subsystems in a tangle of dependencies, rivalries, and sometimes lethal hostilities. Each subsystem is also composed of subgroups and individuals whose desires and needs must be kept in balance, controlled, and, some of the time, met.

Survival is the first imperative of virtually every social system or subsystem. In order to survive, an agency requires funds, staff, clients, administrative structure, and legal authority. To maintain these it must negotiate or compete with other agencies, strive to have good relations with the media, to be viewed favorably in the legislature, to be respected by the professions with which it interacts, to make a good impression on those voluntary organizations that are interested in its field, and to be well thought of by the training institutions that supply it with personnel. In addition, it must recruit and hold several different kinds of staff, each of which has differing expectations and requirements regarding working conditions. The staff makeup of a hospital is a familiar example of these points.

By and large, other interacting subsystems have little or no means for directly viewing the degree to which an agency is actually achieving its stated goals. They and the public, therefore, judge the agency by indicators such as style, reputation, verbal fluency of spokesmen, harmony with current values, and cooperativeness, with the result that the agency strives to make these indicators as impressive as possible. It also strives to create working conditions that will attract and hold staff. The primary goal of care giving, therefore, becomes only one among multiple objectives and is consequently at risk of being obscured.

With these background relationships in mind, we may examine a number of the more dominant specific variables. The first is a common and chronic discrepancy between funds available and cost of achieving the goals envisioned. This comes about because needs are numerous and quality care is expensive. That the problem has been in existence for a great many years is clear from its disastrous role in the great mental hospital movement of the nineteenth century. The advent of universal-service policies has added to its magnitude through increasing the number of people to be seen and treated without a comparable increase in resources. Closely related to the problem of funds is the problem of personnel – the lack of a sufficient number of people who are adequately trained and motivated to fill all the care-giving roles that must be filled if there is to be care of even minimal quality.

A major variable, therefore, in the failure to reach goals on the part of agencies in the mental illness and other care-giving fields is that goals have often been set well beyond the resources in funds and personnel that society at large has so far been willing, or able, to supply in a consistent manner.

Various ripple effects flow from this predicament that further dilute goal achievement. Overload of work, pressure to accomplish impossible tasks, lack of satisfaction in accomplishment, and so on, add up to a considerable accumulation of stressors for individuals on agency staffs, leading them to resign or to do poor work, as will be discussed shortly. Vacancies and rapid turnover in staff, therefore, severely impair the structure and functioning of the services, so that performance is often not even up to the level that would be allowed by the funding. This, in turn, leads to a lowering of standards in hiring policy and the presence of individuals on the staff who are unqualified both technically and psychologically.

The resulting deterioration in the caliber of the staff is apt to be permanent for two reasons. First, potential candidates who have good qualifications for vacant positions are repelled by the prospect of working in a group they perceive to be substandard. Second, the incumbent staff resist admitting to their ranks people with superior professional standing. Those in supervisory positions, in particular, rarely welcome subordinates more highly qualified than themselves. Conversely, individuals with various kinds of technical deficiencies and personality handicaps drift toward these positions and are accepted on the principle that a warm body, even if moribund, is better than no body at all.

The employment of underqualified staff interacts with the agency-survival imperative mentioned earlier. The agency administrators and advisory groups or boards express the survival imperative in their insistence that the clinic or hospital must be kept open at all costs. To do otherwise is to admit a failure that would invite public criticism and that might be politically dangerous. A faulty service is seen as better than none, with the result that those in control placate, appease, and compromise quality in order to keep the agency running.

In such a situation it becomes possible for staff members to hold the service itself hostage, threatening to extinguish it by withdrawal if it is not run according to their liking. Supervision and quality control are then largely abolished, and the unit may pursue goals that are very different from those reflected in its name, its charter, its formal directives, the rhetoric with which it is described, and what people in general expect of it.

Most public-service agencies have, in addition to an operating unit such as a hospital or clinic, a higher office or headquarters in a capital city where policy is made as a result of tradition and of interaction among politicians, top bureaucrats, and health care professionals. It is also common for hospitals, clinics, and especially mental health centers to have a board of advisors or directors who are thought of as "representing the community." They, too, exert directive influence and may contribute to policy.

This troika – operating unit, headquarters, and local board – is liable to serious malfunction at each of its three major interfaces. Operating units have a strong, almost universal, tendency to hold on to and increase as much as possible their independence from the controlling forces of the central office. Equally, the central office strives to maintain and enhance its control. Although variations in popular feeling together with political changes may sway this struggle now one way, now the other, it rarely disappears.

Inasmuch as each contestant has the power to make things exceedingly difficult for the other, the struggle is managed more by indirect strategies – flanking movements and unacknowledged deals – than openly, except during episodes of crisis. As a result, if the struggle becomes intense, both sides may employ half-truths and lies and manipulate rules and regulations rather than abide by them. This, of course, generates a climate of mistrust and may absorb a great deal of an agency's time and energy for matters that have little to do with patient care and that can actually interfere with it.

The relationship between the operating unit and the central administration can be further complicated by differences in their respective guiding sentiments. For instance, the former may be committed to a universal-service policy, whereas the operating unit may retain an ideology based on private and charitable services; or each may have a mixture of these, but different mixtures. Under such circumstances, the staff of a hospital or clinic may exert considerable effort in trying to appear to conform to central-office policy without actually doing so.

It can be argued that a manipulative style of administration matched by covert resistance is the inevitable process of governance, but it can also be argued that its magnitude today, especially in care-giving institutions, is out of hand. The manipulative process can be seen as the result of ethical disarray and lack of commitment to a common goal, which are, in turn, the products of the sociocultural disintegration we have traced to rapid change.

The interface between a board of advisors or directors and the operating unit of an agency has many characteristics similar to those just described. Here again an important part of the dynamic is the hospital or clinic staff's reaching for independence and the countervailing effort by local authorities. From the discussion of communities in Chapter 8, however, it can be anticipated that in many instances a board's capability for coordinated action is exceedingly weak, or else poorly directed and changeable. The spread of differing sentiments within a board is apt to be as great as or greater than that separating central administration and operating unit.

It goes without saying that the interface between board and central administration is fraught with similar problems, as has been illustrated in discussing the double-bind.

Small groups

The translocal networks and subsystems of society, such as the medical profession and care-giving agencies, are of course composed of multiple small groups. The behavior of the larger units, therefore, depends on the small groups' actions as well as on the types of interactions among the larger subsystems just described. By *small group* I mean one in which all members can gather together and in which direct, face-to-face contact is common. A committee, an office staff, a clinical team, and a board of directors are examples. Each such group has assigned tasks to perform and rather characteristic ways of going about the performance of them that affect the goal behavior of the larger social unit of which they form a part.

Let us consider an illustration. When a board or a committee is created, the fact that there are one or more jobs to be done is generally foremost in the minds of the members; this has been called task orientation. As the group settles down to the tasks, however, it finds that ways and means must be developed. Plans must be made and steps toward implementation defined. This, in turn, requires the division of tasks and the assignment and acceptance of roles within the group. Consequently, the managing of interpersonal relationships becomes an essential element in task accomplishment. Even though task achievement is the prime objective, therefore, compromises of various kinds regarding implementation and timing are introduced in order to secure intragroup cooperation and cohesiveness.

Sooner or later in many groups a second phase is reached in which the avoidance of ill feeling, as a means of task accomplishment, takes precedence over the original task. This may be termed *social-emotional orientation*. Its dominance is often not fully recognized by a group's members and might be denied if pointed out.

The social and psychological processes upon which cohesiveness depends are, of course, essential in group effort. Otherwise, there would be no group and so no task accomplishment. The problem is one of balance. The natural history of small groups suggests that this balance is apt to be lost in favor of the social-emotional orientation and at the cost of task accomplishment. The task thus moves down the priority list and goal achievement suffers.

Some activities have built-in correctors that diminish the tendency for social-emotional consideration to become crippling. Winning wars, making profits, and securing votes are of this nature. Errors of inaction in such cases can bring disaster. Service agencies do not, however, have such powerful correctives, and they can run at very inefficient levels for long periods of time unless some spectacular accident occurs that reveals the deficiencies and rouses public indignation.

The tension between social-emotional orientation and task orientation becomes critical when the small group is exposed to stressors. Under these circumstances, it is often the social-emotional orientation that carries the most weight in determining what the group does or does not do. By *stressors* I mean confrontation with decisions that seriously divide the group. This may result from some members' feelings of being threatened by adverse public opinion, political pressure, negative sanctions from hidden constituents, job insecurity, and so forth. We encountered this phenomenon in Chapter 8 when discussing the paralysis of local government in communities.

The response of the small group to the cross-pull between the task and social-emotional orientations may take several different forms:

1   *A task-oriented decision.* The issue is battled out on its merits and within the group's frame of reference. This can happen, but if there is significant conflict within the group it is very apt not to happen.

2   *Denial.* The group maintains that there is no issue and that consequently no decision is required. Even when this is blatantly untrue, the group may nevertheless insist upon it unless outside pressures make such insistence impossible.

3   *Evasion.* This is very similar to denial but is less explicit. Instead, consideration of the issue is postponed, a committee is appointed which never finishes its report, technicalities are discovered that raise the question as to whether it is not really someone else's business, and so on.

If none of these devices work and the issue remains a source of serious intragroup tension, then one can expect structural consequences and sentiments that drastically affect the functioning of the group itself:

4   *Reorganization.* There may be a change of leaders, with the expulsion of those not in favor of the new leaders' point of view. The decision so achieved may be task oriented and lead to an improvement in the group's functioning, but very often it is, instead, dominated by the social-emotional inclinations of one faction in the group and is more a partisan decision than one based on the merits of the case. It may be, therefore, a step that paves the way toward denial or evasion.

5   *Dwindling.* The membership of the group may diminish such that it becomes difficult to muster a quorum or to find people to fill the roles of chairperson, secretary, and so forth. This is likely to come about when the tensions generated by the unresolved confronting issues render the meetings unpleasant. The result is a committee, board, or whatever, that is weak and ineffective in performing its function.

6   *Dissolution.* The group may disappear altogether; this is the logical final stage of dwindling. A new group may be established, but it is often difficult for this to be effective if there has been a long period of dwindling. The image of ineffectiveness attached to the name of the group may prevent the recruiting of capable and highly motivated individuals to a successor organization.

Individual motivation

This review of society at large, agencies, and small groups has highlighted a number of factors that place at risk the accomplishment of goals in many fields of human endeavor, including the care of mental illnesses. Although these factors can be defined and examined in terms of social processes and explained as due to economic, political, sociological, social psychological, and cultural influences, there remains the question of individual motivation. What are the characteristics of human beings that lead them to behave in such a way as to animate so many malfunctional social processes?

The question is one that pertains to much of what has been presented regarding rapid sociocultural change and regarding the structure and functioning of communities, professions, agencies, boards, committees, and clinical teams. We touched upon it early in this chapter by noting that although individuals are extremely dependent on the society of their fellows, they are not in all ways psychologically fitted for the roles their dependence imposes, and I quoted Edgerton's reference to the "wilfullness" that he sees as a part of human behavior in all cultures.

Let us look briefly, therefore, at selected personality processes that help explain these phenomena and that seem to be common to nearly all human beings. The point is that although these processes can become disturbed and lead to socially and psychologically destructive behavior in response to some sets of conditions, in other sets of conditions they can produce behavior that is constructive for the individual and for society.

Some years ago, I attempted to outline a synoptic model of human motivation. It was based partly on research, partly on clinical observation, and partly on a review of literature dealing with motivational theory. The aim was to identify and utilize those concepts upon which the main theorists were agreed. For details and explanation, the reader is referred to the original work.[5] The part that is most relevant here is a list of ten motivational strivings, called essential striving sentiments, that I suggest are universal components of human personality:

1   Physical security
2   Sexual satisfaction

3	Expression of hostility
4	Expression of love
5	Securing of love
6	Securing of recognition
7	Expression of spontaneity
8	Orientation in terms of one's own place in society and the places of others
9	Securing and maintenance of membership in a definite human group
10	Sense of belonging to a moral order and being right in what one does – being in and of a system of values

An individual's role or roles in a medical care-giving agency does not, as a rule, satisfy every one of these major striving patterns, but it is common for several to be involved, such as physical security (salary), obtaining recognition, orientation in terms of one's place in society, membership in a group, and being in and of a system of moral values. If the job role is well designed, some of these vectors of incentive will direct him toward the accomplishment of the agency's goals.

Unfortunately such congruence does not appear in these times to be the common state of affairs. What one finds more often is that the constellation of social structure and shared sentiment that surround individuals in job roles make it necessary for them to do a variety of other things in order to satisfy their essential strivings. Often these other things distract from or run counter to what is needed in order to reach the goals. For example, the striving of individuals for recognition may drive to extremes the struggle of an agency to be independent.

A more structural difficulty is one in which the communication system in the agency is such that word of high-quality goal-directed work does not travel upward very readily. In such a case, gaining recognition may be much more a matter of appearance, pleasing manners, and influential friends. On the other hand, recognition from one's peers in the job situation may be highly contingent on helping to make the conditions of work agreeable to all concerned rather than on technical skill or industrious effort toward goal achievement.

Lack of congruence among the essential striving sentiments that come into play in the work situation can have additional consequences beyond a dilution of effort toward goals. It may, and often does, constitute a conflict that generates severe stressors that lead the individual to react in one of two ways:

1   *Changing the context.* The individual may strive to bring about alterations in the objective situation such as would reduce conflict among the essential strivings that are affected by the work role. This is exceedingly difficult for an individual to accomplish alone, unless the

disharmonies are minor. It is generally the individual who has to give rather than the work environment.

2   *Changing the objectives in the patterns of essential striving.* This response may be summarized by saying that when people find themselves blocked in an essential striving, they seek to maintain the striving by finding a more accessible objective that can serve the same essential purposes in the functioning of their personalities.[6] Taking again the striving for recognition as an example, the objective (approval) may be shifted from supervisor to peers or even outside the work situation altogether to some avocational setting or union activity in which the individual is able to excel. Such a displacement is often at the expense of effort toward the health-care goals of the agency.

When it becomes impossible to relieve severe, conflict-engendered stresses in a work situation by rearranging either the environment or one's essential striving objectives, then a number of other, often nonrational, mechanisms can come into play. Some examples are the following:

1   *Leaving the field.* Evading the task through absenteeism or resignation.
2   *Denial.* Blocking off perception and behaving as if there were no stressors. This may include filling the present with so much to do that there is no time to think about oncoming difficulties.
3   *Reduced activity.* Gloomy apathy and withdrawal into discouraged nonstriving.
4   *Free-floating resentment.* Generally hostile feelings that easily fasten onto scapegoats.
5   *Belief in conspiracy.* The conviction that all difficulties are the result of a deliberate plot directed against one personally.

What I wish to suggest is that human organization can evolve into situations in which their rewards and punishments are so (unwittingly) arranged as to block rather than to foster individual goal-directed behavior, that, further, various kinds of psychological stresses are generated, and finally, that it is these that power many of the malfunctioning societal processes.

Deadlock

The point of departure for this section is the fact that by 1970 the services provided by the Bristol Centre had become the object of a rising tide of adverse criticisms. Although these came from many sources, the most significant of them came from the local doctors. A majority of the physicians in the area expressed alarm for the well-being of their patients and let it be widely known that they had discontinued referring people to the Centre. At one of their meetings I had been asked to attend, I was shown clinical records that were the basis for their concern and their decision to boycott the Centre. The matter was serious primarily because it involved accusations of patient mistreatment, but there were also secondary concerns about the wasting of public funds.

Dealing with this issue was a responsibility of the Board. According to the provincial government's *Policies and Regulations with Regard to Grants-in-Aid,* the Board was to provide "service to patients" and "work as closely and co-operatively as possible with the other personnel and facilities interested in caring for the mentally ill." Heading the list of such personnel and facilities was "the local practicing physician." The document also stated that "The Board is responsible for the recruitment, hiring, work, discipline and discharge of the staff."

The Board never acted on the issue. Although there was a good deal of intense discussion and worrying among members, as an organization it did nothing at all. In this absence of action it provides an example of an organization that disregards one of the main reasons for its existence.

The paralysis, however, was the product not merely of the Board's own functional difficulties, handicapping though these were, but also of the fact that the Board was a component in a web of interactions among a number of other agencies and subsystems. In addition to the staff, these included the Mental Health Administration, the medical subsystem, and the Mental Health Association. The interactions among these units were set in a still more intricate matrix of relationships between each of them and other components of the larger society.[7]

The net effect was a deadlock among parts, the interacting of which would have been necessary in order to bring about a resolution of the patient-care issue. In what follows, I shall attempt to outline some of the main causes of this deadlock. In so doing I shall draw on the concepts, facts, and theories that have been already presented. My aim now, however, is no longer simply a presentation but is instead a demonstration of how the processes interrelate. Taking the patient-care issue as the focal point, I will be concerned with the vectors among the subsystems and, in a sketchier way, with the ties of each to the larger societal and psychological context in which they all existed.

Beginning with the Board's relationship to the staff, there can be little doubt that in the early years the Board established a pattern of being dependent, if not subservient. This fact made it difficult for the Board to reverse itself in order to respond to a situation that called staff performance into question; it required a radical change of orientation and style of interaction. Disbelief, denial, and evasion were easier. The outstanding reasons for the subservience included, first, the difficulties of obtaining and holding staff and, second, the shared sentiment among Board members that their duty was to keep the Centre going in the area and that some kind of center was better than none. These two facts meant that, for the Board, the staff held the existence of the Centre as a hostage.

Another set of factors that put the Board at a disadvantage vis-à-vis the staff were the problems of Board membership recruitment and turnover and the attendant organizational difficulties. These had roots in the fact that the Board was of no great interest to the population of the area served by the Centre, a fact marked by the chronic failure of representatives of local governments to appear at Board meetings. The money given generously by the public during the annual drives of the Mental Health Association, and the appropriations for support voted by most of the local governments of the area, were expressions of belief in the value of the Centre, but not in the value of the Board.

The provincial Mental Health Administration might have intervened and set machinery in motion to evaluate the services being provided by the Centre. The reason it did not was in part because the Board never formally asked for such help. Factors underlying this failure include the patterns of double bind, confrontation, and mistrust that had long existed between the Board and the Administration. As we have seen, the Board and staff of the Centre were united in coping with what many of them regarded as a common enemy. To turn, then, and ask for help from this "enemy" was to run into complex feelings: concern about disloyalty to the staff, a sense of knuckling under to the Administration, damage to pride, and apprehension about exposing the Board to criticism regarding its stewardship during years past.

The Mental Health Administration could, of course, have intervened without waiting for a formal request. To have done so would have been in keeping with an implicit understanding that existed when the Board was founded and with its own public statements about its watchdog duties. The Stirling County Study, as long as it was in charge of the Centre, had held responsibility for the professional standards of the service. When the Board was formed, the understanding was that this particular responsibility passed, not to the lay Board, but to the professionally staffed (even though understaffed) Mental Health Administration. That this was the viewpoint of the Administration, itself, at the time is explicitly stated in a critical review of *More for the Mind* written by a member of the Administration.[8] This article refers to the responsibility of the provincial government for setting and maintaining standards for mental health facilities and warns against the difficulty that arises "when a local board is dominated by some person or group not attuned to modern methods of psychiatry."

The article also states, "Where there is inefficiency and inadequacy at the local level it should be weeded out."

Nevertheless, in the specific patient-care issue that arose at the Centre, there was looking the other way rather than any effort to "weed out." The Administration recoiled like a turtle into its shell. When asked by me about the matter, a representative stated that there had to be a formal written complaint from somebody – if not the Board, then from the doctors, the Mental Health Association, or from patients. In the absence of such a formal document, the Administration felt that if it did anything it would be taking a "considerable risk from a legal point of view." Thus, even though well aware of what the doctors were saying and of other indicators that the Centre was not performing adequately, the Administration took no action. It is difficult to avoid seeing here some repudiation of responsibility and perhaps a parallel to tendencies that have permitted deterioration in many state and provincial mental hospitals.

Whatever the facts about the Administration's actual legal position, it does seem certain that it had many other social and political reasons for being apprehensive about the consequences of intervention. If, for example, no one would put forward a formal complaint, it was reasonable to suppose that there would be equal reticence about supplying information should any kind of inquiry be launched. This would have been awkward, to say the least, and could have left the Administration in difficulties because of the possibility that the staff would have regarded any suggestion of inquiry as damaging to the reputation of its members and would have generated a counterattack in which there would have been support from some Board members, some patients, other individuals in the population, possibly from the provincial association of center staffs, and possibly also from one doctor.

Let us note again that the Administration was a very small organization and that, in addition to the problems of the local Centre, it had to be concerned with the operation of all the other mental health facilities, to provide funds to a number of additional agencies, and to perform consultative functions of various types. Many, if not all, of these centers, hospitals, and other agencies had the same recruiting and related personnel problems as did the Bristol Centre, with the result that the Administration, like the Board, had its enterprises held hostage by their staffs. Thus, there may have been reason for the Administration to fear that if a fracas arose as a result of its attempting to evaluate the Centre, it would be hurt, perhaps badly. Furthermore, it might be that matters would come to light in other areas, some of them of long standing, that were no better than those at Bristol. Thus, again like the Board, the Administration may have been reluctant to initiate a move that could ultimately call into question its stewardship.

Following the advent of Medical Services Insurance in 1969, the total situation was one of instability (again the effect of rapid changes) and the Administration's position was one of vulnerability on many fronts. However reluctant anyone might be to admit it, the question of the well-being of some patients in one locality could well have been an item remote from major concerns.

Because the doctors of the geographic area were the major source of complaints about the service, the local medical association was in a key position to effect improvement. Its members did, indeed, make three attempts to change the situation, but when these failed it took no further action. The first move was for the doctors to talk to the Centre director about their views of the service problems and to encourage him to be more fully a member of the medical group and a sharer in the exchanges of information. The second move was to present the problem to me as head of the Stirling County Study at one of the meetings of the medical association. The hope was that the Stirling County Study would have the influence, if not the authority, to correct the situation. When this expectation proved to be in error, the final move was to ask the chief of psychiatry at Dalhousie University for help. Although he listened sympathetically, he could only point out that he was in no position "to pull your chestnuts out of the fire."

Members of the local medical association also visited the president of the Nova Scotia Medical Society in order to ascertain what the steps might be by which the matter could be brought before the provincial society. Despite a clear statement of what was required and encouragement from the president to go ahead, the physicians decided not to take action along these lines.

The reasons the doctors would not make a formal statement of their concerns to the Board were the same as those which led them to refrain from participation in the Board, namely, resistance to lay control over medical affairs and, in particular, dislike of complaining to lay persons about a doctor. Furthermore, they felt that their obligations to the privacy of their patients meant that they could not present the evidence outside the framework of medically privileged information. This had not been violated in the three moves they did make because all persons involved had been doctors, but this would not be the case if the same information were presented to the Centre Board. Some of the doctors expressed skepticism that the Board could or would do anything even if they overcame their scruples and made a formal complaint, and some were convinced from past experience that certain specific individuals on the Board would be sure to gossip and so could not be trusted with confidential information.

The reasons the doctors would not make a formal complaint to the provincial Mental Health Administration were again related to those that produced withdrawal from the Board, in this case the apprehensions of government control. The doctors' strike in Saskatchewan had been followed in 1970 by a strike of medical specialists in Quebec, and at the time of the issues I am describing, the physicians in Nova Scotia were mobilizing resources to help the Quebec doctors maintain their resistance to control by that provincial government.

Less compelling but still important was the feeling in the minds of some of the local physicians that the Administration, like the Board, would take no effective action even if a formal complaint were made and that, furthermore, certain individuals were not to be trusted with confidences. These views were in part the product of experience and in part an expression of the traditional prejudice of practicing physicians against physicians who "work for the government."

Most of these values, principles, and individual reservations did not apply to the further step which was contemplated by the physicians but not acted upon – namely, taking the issue to the Nova Scotia Medical Society. A minority among the physicians was opposed to exerting this sanction, and so the majority yielded to their wishes rather than risk generating a rift in the group. It happened that the time was particularly inopportune for such a rift because a group practice was being formed in Bristol and the doctors strongly wished for goodwill and cooperation among all members of the local medical subsystem.

I have mentioned in connection with the Board and the Mental Health Administration my impression that an inhibiting factor was apprehension lest an inquiry raise questions about stewardship. A possible counterpart of this in the medical group was the feeling that few, if any, doctors were so consistently excellent in their practice as to be above criticism and that if any inquiry and evaluation of the Centre were carried out, it might stimulate retaliation, or at least set a dangerous precedent.

Before leaving the medical subsystem, it is worth noting that although the doctors failed in the end to carry out effective action, they displayed much more concern about patient care than did the laymen of the citizen Board who were supposed to "represent" the Centre's clients. I point this out in view of the accusations that are commonly leveled at physicians that they are self-serving. It would seem that when a lay group is exposed to an analogous cross-pull of influences, it may very well do no better in protecting the interests of those it is supposed to represent. In the case we are discussing, the doctors' greater concern appeared to stem from their direct personal contact with suffering individuals. They saw the harmful consequences of the Centre's actions concretely, whereas the Board saw them only abstractly and, hence, could more easily dismiss, deny, or rationalize them.

The Mental Health Association might have played an active role with regard to the functioning of the Centre, and it could have issued a formal request to the Mental Health Administration for inquiry and evaluation. Most of the reasons it did not do so have been covered in discussing the Board, for, as we have seen, the Board was largely made up of the Bristol and Kingston Mental Health Associations. The aims of these organizations were educational and promotional. Like all such associations, their energy was devoted to creating a climate of public opinion favorable to fund raising and mobilizing political force toward expanding and developing mental health services. It was understandable, therefore, that local as well as provincial mental health associations were reluctant to take the initiative in demanding that an inquiry take place. The result might have been a negative picture of one of the enterprises (the Centre) they had been strongly supporting and for which they had persuaded people to give a considerable sum of money. The long-range goals for achieving public benefit in terms of mental health services could seem to dictate that it would be better to avoid this particular issue if at all possible.

Inasmuch as lack of communication is often cited as the major source of difficulty in human relations, let us note that, in this case, lack of information about the problem was not an obstacle. The deficiency in formal communications was secondary to the other factors outlined. Individuals among the members of the Board, the staff, the Mental Health Administration, the local medical association, the mental health associations, and the Stirling County Study did talk informally with each other. There were, of course, numerous misperceptions, denials, and so forth, due to the social roles, network positions, and sentiment systems of the various persons concerned, but the flow of information per se was not greatly inhibited by refusals to use formal channels.

Although the Stirling County Study was not one of the components of the deadlock, it was nevertheless indirectly involved, and a few words should be said about this. During the school issue, as the reader may recall, the members of the Study endeavored to persuade the Centre to abstain from active participation in the conflict. This was ineffective and resulted in the staff breaking their connections with the Study. Under these circumstances, it seemed to me and the other members of the Study that pressing the matter would be destructive, and so we discontinued further effort to interfere with what the staff wanted to do.

When the issue of patient care arose and the doctors came to me as head of the Stirling County Study for help, I pointed out to them that since 1961, as a nonvoting member of the Board, my role had been advisory only. Within that framework, however, I undertook to discuss the matter with the Centre staff and to seek cooperation in reviewing the difficulties perceived by the physicians. When the staff refused, I tried again at the Board level and sought to have a committee appointed that would be composed of the public health officers (ex-officio Board members) and three other physicians who would sit down with the director in a spirit of mutual respect and helpfulness and explore the nature of the problems and their possible solutions. The committee was authorized by the Board but was never appointed by the chairperson. I then had a number of discussions with the Mental Health Administration. The position taken there, as I have reported above, was that no action could be initiated unless a formal complaint were lodged. Thus, although the Study felt its way around the circle of the deadlock, it could not find a way to break it.

Pervading all sections of the deadlock and their interrelationships was the crisis triggered by the school issue. It is possible that under "routine conditions," the deadlock might in time have been loosened, very likely through informal procedures, and resulted in some evaluation of the Centre's activities, managed with due regard for both patients and staff and without the glare of media reporting. Under the conditions that existed, however, the crisis climate heightened polarization, creating in some groups a determination to "win" rather than to look at facts and issues and in others an immobility inspired by self-preservation.

The reader will recall that the school issue was precipitated by the dismissal of a teacher. It did not take much imagination to see the same drama reenacted with the Centre as the focus, should its Board appear to censure a member of the staff. The forces opposed to the school administration gave every appearance of being on the lookout for a new martyr. Although it is doubtful that any of the Board or town leaders had read Kornhauser, many felt in their bones that in a new controversy, they would indeed lose to "those elements in the community who do not have power," and for the very reasons Kornhauser pointed out.[9] The school issue had shown how hard and long and with what zest those "who do not have power" could work as attackers. Particularly effective in mobilizing support and weakening opposition was the charge of conspiracy. As Kornhauser says, it was "crucial." It appealed to what people with grievances and grudges of all kinds were glad to believe, and it made those in positions of responsibility anxious to show that they were not really engaged in conspiracy. The latter often took the form of silence and refusal to oppose the attackers.

It was very clear that charges of conspiracy would again be employed if steps were taken to look into the quality of the service being supplied by the Centre staff. Such charges were, in fact, employed when Board members, the Stirling County Study, and others tried to dissuade the staff from participation in the school issue. They were raised again in response to the physicians' expressions of concern about patients and when the Stirling County Study and Board members suggested that the whole matter might be resolved if a committee of the Board and the staff were to join in a cooperative look at the facts. The staff expressed the view that any question raising was tantamount to an accusation and was the product of a conspiratorial effort by "powerful" individuals and agencies in Bristol who had been offended by the staff's behavior in the school issue and who did not like its siding with "the little people" against those in power.

This, then, was the deadlock of inaction in which the subsystems were bound. All participants were involved in the pursuit of objectives that took precedence over patient care. As the deadlock moved on through time, the doctors' complaints about patient care also continued. Matters stood thus when our reporting period ended on March 31, 1972.

11 Approaches to action

Before turning to a discussion of possibilities for action, I shall attempt to summarize the main points that have been derived from our case study of the Bristol Mental Health Centre. The order of topics in the recapitulation is in reverse order of that previously given. Instead of beginning with mental illnesses and moving out from them to relevant societal processes and eventually to society at large, I shall begin with some salient characteristics of Western society and then move step by step to the problems of controlling mental illnesses in this context. The reason for the reversal is to emphasize the reciprocal nature of the interconnections; influence does not flow in one direction only.

Recapitulation

Society at large

Two features of modern society in North America, as in much of the rest of the world, have had and continue to have a profound effect on its institutions and organizations:

1   *Accelerating change* in the structure of subsystems of society and in the shared sentiments (values, beliefs, and perceptions of reality) that make up the guidelines of human orientation and human conduct.
2   *Social-cultural disintegration* stemming from the accelerating change and consisting of the breakdown of functioning within and between the various subsystems. This results because the rate of social change exceeds the rate of adaptation to it.

Agencies concerned with the care of mental illnesses are among the institutions and organizations affected, as are most of the other agencies with which they interact. The impact of accelerating change and social disintegration weakens the capacity to overcome the four barriers discussed in Chapter 2 (and summarized later in this chapter) and hinders the achievement of goals.

The conditions of life in a society that is far gone toward disintegration are psychologically stressful for most of the individuals who experience them. Stress may become so severe as to inflate the rates of at least some kinds of mental illnesses. Thus, social disintegration appears to increase the need for care of mental illnesses and at the same time to decrease the means for meeting this need due to malfunction of organizations. In any event, there is epidemiological data to show that, whatever the cause, the prevalence rates for many, if not all, kinds of mental illnesses are higher in severely disintegrating societies than in those that are socially and culturally integrated.[1]

Communities

The idea of community as a social unit of major significance has long been associated with the mental health movement. Although the meaning of the word *community* is exceedingly loose, it generally implies people living in a geographically defined area who have some sense of identity with the area and each other, who have some capability for self-determination, and who are competent in the management of local affairs.

Faith in community competence for self-management has led many of those in the mental health movement to plan and think in terms of an ideal model that has not closely matched the realities revealed in numerous community studies. Further, during the third quarter of the present century, the discrepancies between the ideal and reality have increased rather than decreased, resulting in many disappointing, and some disastrous, outcomes of policymaking and planning (see section on communityism later in this chapter).

There can be little doubt that clusters of people that can be defined as competent, self-managing communities do exist, but their numbers are not great, and the trends over the last half century, continuing into the present, are not in their favor. Many geographically defined populations are not so much communities as crossroads for "regional and national networks of goods, services, and institutional behavior patterns and control, with little locally initiated and locally determined action."[2] The attributes of population clusters that work against their abilities to function in terms of participatory democracy and self-management may be summarized along two main dimensions, each with several major subsets:

1   *A social structure that weakens rather than supports the community ideal*
     a   Variability of boundaries according to purpose (schools, health, etc.). As a result, it is often difficult to say where the limits of a community lie and, hence, to define it.

b   Mobility of population. This produces a turnover among leaders and a general reduction of concern about local affairs; long-range planning, in particular, is adversely affected.

c   Control of local affairs by outside powers. Major decisions that affect education, health, welfare, and the economy are made outside the local area. Further, those decisions that are made by local leaders, boards, and committees are subject to strong, sometimes covert, influences from people and institutions beyond the limits of the local area – "hidden constituencies."

d   Special-interest groups with a shallow sociopolitical power base. The shallow base derives in part from the above three attributes and in part from the quality of having a special interest. As a result, organizations such as mental health associations, although they may be able to raise money, may not represent "the people" or have the backing necessary for a sustained impact on local affairs. In fact, their single-minded struggles, by disregarding other local needs and issues, may undermine rather than foster participatory democracy.

2   *Shared patterns of sentiment that weaken rather than support the community ideal*

a   General inertia toward participation in local affairs. There may be goodwill toward good works, but at the same time there is commonly an unwillingness to become actively engaged.

b   Weak sense of community identity and of belonging together. This, of course, is much under the influence of population mobility and uncertain boundaries.

c   A desire to avoid trouble in interpersonal relations at all costs. Most people do not wish to enter controversies, even if, thereby, they overlook issues that are important for the common good.

d   Disparagement of the local area. Widespread in smaller population clusters, but also found in some larger ones, this sentiment often appears as a rationalization for inertia.

e   The spread of cosmopolitan sentiments to smaller populations. Such sentiments include a dominance of instrumental rather than humanistic attitudes toward most other people, together with an expectation of sooner or later moving on and, hence, a lack of feeling for local roots.

These two dimensions (structure and shared sentiments) of incompatibility with the ideal community model, together with their subsets, are highly interactive. As a result, many geographically definable populations are to a large extent devoid of the kind of autonomy and competence visualized in plans for decentralization and the turning of responsibility for mental health care over to communities.

Finally, let us note that communities are subject to crises in which nonrational states of mind and the consequent activities disrupt whatever structure exists, produce changes in shared sentiments, and set people against each other. These behaviors are undoubtedly often in part a reaction to stressful conditions, but that does not mean that they are liable to produce improved self-management and coping abilities on the part of a population. Conversely, the disruptive effects may last for a considerable period of time, forcing the intervention of various kinds of agencies from outside the area.

Although the period of the late sixties and early seventies was a time when there was an epidemic of crises, it is evident that human society has a long history of such events. It seems likely, furthermore, that, because of the emotions aroused by social and cultural disintegration, the risk of crises is proportional to the disintegrative forces at work.

The medical profession

During the third quarter of the present century, the medical profession was under pressure to shift from private-practice and charitable models of service to a universal model operating on the principle that every individual is entitled to medical care "without hindrance of any kind."[3] The consequences may be summed up as follows:

1   *Organizational and ideational ambiguities* regarding the conduct of medical affairs. Reasonable, unreasonable, and impossible demands were made of physicians, and they responded with a mix of adaptation, resistance, and confusion. Thus, the medical subsystem experienced a certain amount of disorganization, and its members felt a considerable degree of emotional distress.
2   *Protection of working conditions.* This was a main response to the pressure for change. It took shape in a closing of ranks, resisting government control, and trying to prevent the intrusion of laymen into what was conceived of as medical affairs.
3   *Separation from community mental health.* This was in line with the above protection of working conditions. Psychiatry itself was not repudiated but rather was invited to join in the solidarity of the medical subsystem. What was repudiated was the notion of a medical-psychiatric service being controlled by a consortium of government officials, local laymen, and nonmedical professionals.

Care-giving agencies

Care-giving agencies comprise another subsystem of society that, like the medical profession, is apt to be present in any given community or population cluster and that, at the same time, belongs to a much larger network and is therefore subject to influences from the outside that can interfere with the ability (and freedom) to serve local clients. The result is behavior that on occasion seems calculated to do everything except fulfill the goals that are supposedly the basis for the agencies' existence. The complex of reasons for such malfunction can be summed up as follows:

1   *Survival* as the first imperative of agency existence. This means a continuing stream of internal and external adjustments and adaptations many of which are far removed from, and may even run counter to, the proper care of clients.

2   Chronic or recurrent *inadequacy of resources*. This discrepancy between goals and resources has two interlocked forms: money and competent personnel. It springs from the fact that society is more willing to authorize than to pay for humane goals, especially in the mental illness field. Two consequences are notable: (a) the imposition of many stresses on those who work in care-giving agencies, which produces emotional reactions and defenses that may further defeat the achievement of care-giving goals; (b) still greater deterioration of resources – in other words, a downward spiral whereby the reality and reputation of bad performance discourages funding and drives away competent personnel.

3   *Misalignment of rewards and goal achievement*. This means that the individuals employed in an agency are more apt to be rewarded for behaviors that bear on agency defense and survival than for high-quality care giving and cooperation with other agencies.

Conditions generated by rapid change and social disintegration in the larger society augment the problems of survival and funding and disconnect still more the reward system from quality performance. As social disintegration progresses, rewards of all kinds become progressively more arbitrary, impulse-ridden and, unpredictable.[4]

Small groups

Much of the decision making in the subsystems of society is conducted in small groups such as committees and boards. Such is the case in communities, professions, agencies, and various levels of government. It follows, therefore, that the behavior characteristic of small groups has consequences affecting how the larger subsystems perform. Like all other organizations, small groups are adversely affected by rapid rates of turnover in membership. Beyond this, however, they have two major characteristics that are more particularly their own:

1   *The tendency for a social-emotional orientation to supersede task orientation*. Because they are composed of individuals who come to

know one another, small groups require a positive social-emotional climate in order to function. Unless there are specific corrective factors at work, however, there is a tendency for the social-emotional orientation to obscure the concern for task accomplishment, with negative consequences for goal achievement. People frown on "rate busters" – that is, individuals who set task achievement ahead of group loyalty.

2   *Responses to stress that deflect attention from tasks.* Social change and social disintegration often impose conditions of exceptional stress on small groups, and, when they do, finding relief from the stress is apt to take precedence over accomplishing tasks or goals. This is particularly likely to be the case when task accomplishment is inseparable from the stress-causing situation. Under such circumstances, the small group is likely to manifest various combinations of denial, evasion, and reorganization, accompanied by goal changes, or else the group may dwindle and disappear.

The mental illness field

There are four major barriers to effective mental health care that consist of social and psychological factors intrinsic to the field:

1   The extreme *heterogeneity* of mental illnesses combined with a common tendency of people generally to treat them as if they were one. This *lump thinking* obscures the criteria for priorities, disturbs the accurate perception of innumerable problems and issues, and clouds policymaking and management.

2   The *strong emotions* generated by mental illnesses and even by the notion of mental illnesses. These lead to many nonrational and emotional lines of action and greatly magnify the problems created by barrier one. They render the field highly susceptible to magical thinking, dogmas, ideologies, mysticism, and transient fashions that often swing across wide extremes. Goals and goal seeking thus become highly unstable and liable to unpredictable shifts.

3   The *insufficient use of science.* This springs from the combination of barriers one and two with the result that the resources of science have not been brought sufficiently to bear on the development of a coherent and widely accepted frame of reference. The consequences have been deleterious for policy formation and planning and for public understanding. With some exceptions, a scientific perspective has not been an antidote to magical thinking and has not had a sustained influence on understanding, controlling, and preventing mental illnesses.

4   The *combination of an extraordinarily large number of goals with a very small number of clearly understood and widely accepted priorities.* The result is lack of coordination and scattering of effort that can be summed up as the Lord Ronald syndrome (see Chapter 2). Cycles of enthusiasm bloom and then become blighted, with much damage to

the care of mentally ill individuals (illustrations of this tendency can be found in Chapters 3, 5, and 10).

The third quarter of the present century was a time when the growing mental health movement revealed many flaws stemming from its own Lord Ronald tendencies, flaws that eroded and crippled its nascent organizations. Acting on these flaws was a burst of new ideas and activities from within and without the movement, many of which were incompatible, hostile, and intensely competitive with one another. Old goals and old organizations were weakened or swept away, and adequate replacements failed to emerge.

As has been related, rapid change is now the most steadfast characteristic of society at large. It is commonly accompanied by institutional disintegration and malfunctioning, the disruption of shared sentiments, and the psychological disturbance of individuals caught up in these processes. What clinicians and other mental health professionals can do about this state of affairs, within the framework of their professions, may be very little. To a major extent, the turbulence of the larger societal context is something that has to be endured – like stormy weather.

But not altogether. Even stormy weather is better taken into account than ignored.

Approaches to action

The first point in approaching action is the importance of *recognition*. The reality and character of the barriers to better care for mental illnesses must become widely known and understood if there is to be a sustained advance upon them. The hindrances must be seen for what they are – not separate, occasional, or incidental difficulties, but a tough fabric of closely interwoven recalcitrant psychological, social, economic, and cultural processes of long standing. Disregard of them leads to poor planning, and poor planning, as the President's Commission observed, "can confuse priorities, divert administrative energies and waste money. The victims of this disarray are the people who need care, the local programs and agencies which provide it, and the taxpayers who must pay for it . . . [T]he planning process which now exists is not adequate to the task."[5]

Recognition of the nature of the confronting problems will make clear the need for a *reassessment* of the kind of information and the kind of thinking commonly employed in policymaking, planning, and delivery of service. Such reassessment should, in turn, cause a drastic reduction in the accepted wisdom about mental illnesses by revealing it to contain many unsubstantiated beliefs, mistaken assumptions, and mischievous half truths.

Mr. Justice Holmes once observed that all life is an experiment and, further, that "Every year if not every day we have to wager our salvation upon some prophecy based upon imperfect knowledge."[6] This wise saying needs to be balanced by Josh Billing's view (paraphrased here) that "it ain't so much ignorance that hurts folks as knowing so dern many things that ain't so." If we wish to improve our performances, whether as individuals or as a society, it behooves us to struggle continuously and relentlessly to reduce as much as possible the proportion of error in the information on which we base our decisions.

Although it may be true, as many critics of psychiatry and psychology aver, that we know more than we practice, it is even more true that we practice and advocate far more than we know. A major step toward better understanding, therefore, is to identify the speculations and fabrications that hide the holes in our knowledge.

After reduction and cleaning, the veridical residue must then be applied. *Application* is not necessarily transitive; it may be orientative and result in skeptical caution and a wise ability to take a long-range rather than a short-range view and to stay off careening bandwagons. But it also includes direct action in the design of workable priorities, the formation of public policy, the development of programs, and education that is based on information rather than ideologies. Perhaps we are ready for an updated version of Adolf Meyer's "commonsense psychiatry" and its employment by political leaders, administrators, teachers, students, clinicians, voluntary-association members, and those who work in the media.[7]

Parallel with application, and hard on the heels of reassessment and the reduction of spurious information, there must come expansion of knowledge through *scientific research*. When one thinks of mental illnesses and research together, it is generally in terms of discovering causes and cures. Social psychiatry, for example, has been largely concerned with the role of social and cultural factors in the origin, course, and outcome of disorders and in the treatment and prevention of disorders. The importance of etiological, therapeutic, and preventive research goes without saying, but it is important also to note that there are other objectives that demand attention. The nature of, and the reasons for, the four barriers to effective care is one example. The numerous social processes that affect the functioning of mental illness services constitute another. These are research areas that have not, as yet, been sufficiently developed, and they suggest an expansion of the definition of social psychiatry.

Recognition, reassessment, research, and application are the key ideas in the discussion of approaches to action that follows.

Education and training

Education and training are essential for developing the seedbeds in which recognition, reassessment, research, and application can flourish. The experience of the present study suggests the desirability of programs at many levels from early preparation to advanced study and continuing education. The professions active in the care of mental illnesses should be the primary focus, but, because what they can do by themselves is limited, the focus must be extended to include people in management, law, government, and the media.

It may also be suggested that many of the compartmentalizations that now exist should be softened and turned into boundaries for the transaction of exchange rather than maintained as walls that resist cross-communication. The kind of walls I have in mind are those that lie between practice and research, between academic institutions and care-giving agencies, between central administration and operating units, and among the various professions and disciplines that make up the mental illness field or that, like the law, markedly influence its policies and patterns of action.

This might be accomplished by more rotations within training programs than currently exist. For example, many perduring problems might be diminished if it were standard procedure for clinics and centers that provide services to have regular research and training responsibilities as well. This could help make practitioners more interested in and comprehending of scientific investigation and therefore more apt to utilize the results with discernment. It is possible also that cooperation among the professions and disciplines might be enhanced if psychiatrists, psychologists, social workers, nurses, and others received selected parts of their training together. This could apply particularly to learning about the sociocultural processes that affect the distribution and care of mental illnesses in populations, learning about processes that play a major part in the behavior of small groups such as clinics, hospitals, centers, and boards, and learning about research methods and how to utilize research results. Much of the instruction could be based on case examples. In addition to rotation of trainees, such programs should also include joint appointments for trainees and exchanges with academic institutions.

Careful planning, staging, and management would of course be necessary or the result could be an increase rather than a decrease in malfunctioning. An essential point would be to have the research and training activities of agency members defined as part of their jobs and not considered merely "something on the side." With good management, the presence of training and research in agencies would serve as a stimulation to continuous updating of knowledge, and it could help in attracting competent personnel, both of which would be beneficial to the quality of services.

The content of what should be taught in programs for education and training must always have the essentials for professional competence at its core. A clinician, for instance, must be thoroughly versed in diagnosis and treatment. These are minimal requirements, however, and not sufficient for improving the care of mental illnesses and bringing about greater recognition, reassessment, research, and application.

The kinds of additional topics that are important have been adumbrated in the preceding chapters and outlined again at the beginning of this chapter. Their full development for educational and training purposes is, of course, a large undertaking, and one beyond the scope of this book. It is possible, however, to make a number of suggestions regarding areas of emphasis for both instruction and action. These now follow, beginning with rather general matters of orientation and moving toward those that are more specific and programmatic.

Individualism

Emphasizing the individual, while at the same time failing to pay attention to the social setting of which that individual is a part, is an occupational bias found in many clinicians, whether psychiatrists or psychologists. From beginning to end it was evident in the functioning of the Bristol Mental Health Centre despite the presence and conscious efforts of the Stirling County Study. It was most obvious in the Centre's relationships with the Bristol schools, but it permeated most other relationships as well. It set severe limits on the staff's ability to perform as an exemplar of social psychiatry in action and, in some instances, produced results that were destructive.

The larger picture across North America reveals many similar instances, of which the headlong character of deinstitutionalization has been one of the most serious. There have been others, however, some with origins that go back many years. Two examples are the following.

Some time ago, psychiatrists and clinical psychologists began to point out that mothers could harm children by bringing about too much repression of natural drives. In time, a major attack on mothers was under way, one which blamed them for whatever disturbances occurred in their children during later life. The notion was individual centered, with better mental health for "the child" as its impeccable goal. But what were its effects on mothers and, therefore, on relationships among mothers, fathers, and older children? In short, what were its effects on the family as a social institution?

Something similar has happened with regard to schools. Stereotypes came into being that pictured the teacher as the enemy of the child and the school administration as the enemy of both. The issue was not so much good education as the psychological evils of suppressing natural feelings and free expression. Again we may ask whether the input from psychiatrists and psychologists was the result of tunnel vision and was overdone, and also whether it played a significant part in the current widespread demoralization of teachers and in the semidisintegration now evident in numerous educational systems, neither of which can be very good for "the child."

These observations are not intended to deny some truth in the theories of repression, nor to advocate the hiding of difficult truths lest they disturb the social status quo. But they are a plea for better recognition by clinicians of the interrelationships between individual behavior and the functioning of social institutions upon which the well-being of innumerable individuals depends. Such understanding might then be applied to the formulation of better balanced plans for constructive action.

The advent of a policy of universal medical service in Canada and its approach in the United States increases the risks that attend the type of individualism I have defined. This is because under universal service the care-giving systems have responsibility not only for those who are ill now but also for those who will become ill next year or later. Consequently, the not-yet-ill have to be given as much consideration as the ill. But whatever is done for the ill must not be of such a character as to add health hazards and increase the illness risk for the not-yet-ill. In this framework, mothers, teachers, administrators, and their sisters and their cousins and their aunts, together with all other kinds of persons, must be taken into account in health-care thinking just as much as the individual who is, at any given moment, under treatment.

This is not a new conception, and working models already exist. Until recently, however, it has been applied only to certain segments of the population such as the military, where the medical service has the health of all personnel as its responsibility, not just that of those who are currently ill.

We must modify a tendency we mental illness professionals have to fight blindly on behalf of patients against their environment. We must recognize that for any human being the environment is largely other people who are, themselves, at risk for developing mental illnesses, or who are already coping with such disorders as best they may even if not yet designated patients. At any given moment, some 20 percent of the population have mental illnesses of some kind whether they are being treated or not.

But the advent of universal service means more than this. It means that the operating components of society – institutions and organizations – require from social planners understanding and recognition of what makes them function well or badly. It also means understanding what the consequences are, when they function badly, for those people who compose them or are affected by them.

Many of the counterculture and "me generation" ideas discussed in Chapter 5 borrowed heavily from individualistic themes furnished by psychiatry such as, for instance, the importance of freedom from repression. These were turned against us in the blooming of antipsychiatry not only by youth groups and cultists but also by other mental health professionals and by lawyers defending the rights of the individual. We discovered that we, the psychiatry subsystem, were being hoisted by a petard that we had helped assemble. As a profession and therefore a social institution, we were being blown up by individualistic concepts that failed to take into account their consequences for social institutions – very much as had happened to families and schools.

To restate this theme in a few words, the individualistic orientation of our clinical professions needs to be enriched with understanding of societal systems.

Communityism

By communityism, I mean the kind of indiscriminate lump thinking about, and uncritical faith in, the vague but ideal model of communities outlined in Chapter 8 that is so commonly suffused with considerable emotion. This notion of *community* was introduced into a psychiatry that was not prepared to give it adequate evaluation.[8] This is evident in *More for the Mind*, published in 1963, which in its call for decentralization of mental health services implies unqualified confidence in "the local community."[9]

The beginnings of communityism, however, were much earlier. From 1946 onward, members of the mental health leadership in the United

States became more and more committed to the concept of *community care*.[10] This trend resulted in the launching (also in 1963) of a program intended to create 2,000 "community" centers that would enable the mentally ill to be "successfully and quickly treated in their communities."

But from the 1920s onward, a succession of community studies had been conducted in the United States and Canada in urban, suburban, and rural areas. A selection of the major works, ranging from *Middletown* to *Crestwood Heights,* were reviewed and the results published in 1960 under a significant title, *The Eclipse of Community.* The contrast between these findings and the unquestioning belief in the capacities of communities on the part of the mental health movement is very striking. *The Eclipse of Community* speaks of fading local leadership, of the dominance of outside industrial, bureaucratic, and urban powers, and of the sentiments that show "the successive weakening of national ties, regional ties, community ties, neighborhood ties, family ties and finally, ties to a coherent image of oneself."[11] It further adds that "heightened functional dependence and diminished loyalties appear in most sociological diagnoses of our time." The essay touches on many of the phenomena observed in the course of our case study of the Centre and on many of the points made in discussing the community concept in Chapter 8.

The implication of all this is obvious: Communityism builds on sand – that is, it creates projects and programs that are at high risk of faltering and betraying expectations because they stand on false assumptions. The President's Commission of 1978 is more discriminating than many of its predecessors in that it recognizes the failure of numerous community programs as due to lack of the necessary services and responsiveness. Its tone remains, however, too confident in what communities can do. It also fails to sort out those societal processes that are or could be under local control from those that are most often transcommunity in character. Thus, it mixes together "churches and synagogues, schools, employers, unions, and civic clubs and voluntary organizations." It also speaks of Alcoholics Anonymous, Foster Grandparents, and "the civil and criminal justice system."[12]

All of these, of course, have impacts on individuals at local levels, but there is great variation among them in the degree to which they are susceptible to local influence directed at changing how they interact with mental health or illness problems. Many of them, because they are parts of transcommunity networks, are more apt to respond, if at all, at higher levels in their organization than a community branch.

In sum, communityism encompasses incomplete and false perceptions about the nature of society that are widely and approvingly held in North America. The people who formed and led the community mental health center movement participated in this orientation, and in the associated shared sentiments, without critical examination of the facts. They have, as a consequence, been let down in their expectations.

In considering these matters, however, it is important not to react by a swing from one erroneous extreme to another – from too much confidence to rejecting the whole idea of community and local participation. The appropriate reaction is to develop more sophisticated concepts that apprehend the interplay of communities and transcommunity networks. Only then can the way be opened for understanding the synergies possible between communities and transcommunity systems and for basing policy on such knowledge. Some suggestions toward this end follow.

Modification of individualism. A forward step would be modifying through education the individualism discussed in the previous section that limits the clinician's ability to think in social-process terms. Another would be the improvement of communication among the disciplines so that the work of those researchers who have conducted empirical studies of social processes are known to clinicians and planners of clinical services.

Part of the problem, of course, is the magnitude of contemporary knowledge. At whatever point one stands, knowledge stretches out of sight in all directions, and there are always elements below the horizon that would be of significance to one's work if only one knew about them. Added to this is the fact that the way knowledge is organized into disciplines, for teaching and research, effectively reduces communication to a few conventional channels. Even these, unfortunately, have been further reduced during the last thirty years as many of the social sciences withdrew from interdisciplinary activities. Concomitant with this was a loss of interest in the study of communities.

A further obstacle is that some, and perhaps many, clinicians think of scientific research as having only two principal methods: (a) experiment; and (b) reasoned theory building from postulates that are assumed to be general truths, following the model exemplified by Freud. In making this dichotomy, clinicians overlook the existence of epidemiology in their own field and also, in more general terms, the existence of a third scientific method that produces descriptions and comparisons (often empirical) based on quantitative data. Geology, oceanography, and astronomy are examples of branches of science that rely heavily on such methods.

Because of their dichotomous orientation toward science, many psychiatrists and psychologists conclude that because sociology and anthropology are obviously not primarily experimental in their methods, they must be regarded as builders of theory from postulates. Indeed, it is interesting to note that there are parallels in mode of thinking to be found among the leaders of psychodynamic thought (such as Freud, Adler, Jung, Sullivan, Fromm, Erikson, and Horney) and those economists, sociologists, and anthropologists most apt to be known to clinicians (such as Marx, Weber, Veblen, G. H. Mead, Parsons, Benedict, M. Mead, Goffman, Riesman, and Lévi-Strauss).

Because they perceive sociology and anthropology to be theoretical and analytical disciplines, psychiatrists and psychologists overlook the existence of empirical studies and quantitative investigations of hypotheses. Works such as those of Stouffer, Warner, Suchman, Chappel, Lazersfeld, Sol Levine, Robin Williams, and Ted Graves are hardly known to them.[13] As a result, sociology and anthropology are seen not as fields that contain a growing body of conclusions based on quantitative data but rather as fields made up of speculative theories (something like psychodynamics), each with its passionate adherents. Important knowledge that is well founded in observation is therefore likely to be unrecognized, as I shall point out presently in further discussing the community mental health center movement.

American sociologists have contributed to this state of affairs by losing much of the interest they once had in empirical studies and replacing it with an emphasis on postulate-based theories. At mid-century, American sociology was outstanding for its emphasis on empirical research and stood in marked contrast to European sociology, which had always contained a strong element of political philosophy. The diminution of empiricism and hypothesis checking has helped obscure sociology's factual achievements and its potential usefulness in the kinds of problems under discussion.

Factual studies about the care of mental illnesses. It would be helpful now if there were a new wave of factual studies oriented by questions arising from efforts to provide care for mental illnesses. From the thirties to the mid-fifties, the problem of community acceptance of innovation was a major topic of investigation, especially with reference to self-help, self-government, and other programs concerned with the common good. They arose from such issues as how to control soil erosion and how to adopt new methods in crop production and also from various projects aimed at improving housing, nutrition, and health. The work was sponsored by agencies in the U.S. Department of Agriculture, the Bureau of Indian Affairs, and various state governments and by private foundations, particularly the Russell Sage Foundation. Much was learned about pitfalls in community planning and some about principles and methods that could increase chances of success. The work, however, was far removed physically, intellectually, and bureaucratically from those engaged in developing the community mental health program.

The political process. Another step would be to find ways and means for dealing with simplistic notions generated by political processes. Like *mental health,* the word *community* arouses a favorable response, from the public, from the media, and from many elected representatives. Nearly everyone who tries to convince people about a program finds that initial success is more apt to occur by building on what people think they know rather than attempting their reeducation. This means operating with stereotypes, conventional wisdom, and prevailing opinions, and it discourages investigations that might call such ideas into question or require that they be modified. For the long-run outcome, however, this can be exceedingly costly.

As Foley has reported, the creation of the community mental health center program in the United States and the securing of the necessary legislation was the work of a coalition composed of people in the federal government, in Congress, in the American Psychiatric Association and other professional associations, and in the National Mental Health Association. This coalition turned away from the goal of improving the state hospitals (which was part of the recommendation of the Joint Commission on Mental Illness and Health) and chose instead to emphasize exclusively the Joint Commission's companion goal of care in the community.[14] Once accepted, the idea became a sentiment that was not only vital to the (social-emotional) cohesiveness of the coalition but was also central to building the political support necessary to secure legislative approval and presidential backing. It was politically unacceptable from that point onward, therefore, to be concerned with scientific truth and to let community care seem to be what it actually was and still is – full of serious unresolved problems. It was no longer acceptable to point out that state and provincial hospitals had come into existence originally because community care had been so atrocious[15] or to ask for evidence that a better outcome could be expected now. Nor was it acceptable to pay attention to the fact that, as recently as the 1930s, enormous numbers of "communities" had failed to cope with their welfare problems, but left matters to state and federal governments, and to inquire what lessons might be had from these experiences.

If someone had wanted to run a series of research projects in order to assess communities and explore for feasible models of community care, he would have threatened the coalition on at least two counts: first, the danger of providing material with which the opponents of the program could attack it; and second, the danger of delay that would lose the moment when Congress and the public seemed ready to accept the program. As with the great mental hospital movement over a hundred years before, energy and attention were on what had to be done to start the programs, not on issues of long-range feasibility.[16]

The coalition was exceedingly well grounded in clinical knowledge, and it was fully aware of the neglect and mistreatment to which many persons with mental illnesses were subjected. The members were distinguished for their humanity, as well as for their political astuteness. They were also scientific in part of their orientation and fostered the gathering and utilization of vast amounts of information pertaining to the practices and concepts of mental illness care, as can be seen in the ten volumes produced by the joint commission. Conspicuously absent, however, were studies of community structure and functioning concerned with delineating the problems that would have to be solved if the community-care program were to be something better than the state hospitals.[17]

It is an interesting fact that, despite their individualism, clinicians can still be well acquainted with the political process. What they often do not realize, however, is that it is only a narrow and somewhat superficial segment in the working of social systems. It pertains to the distribution and rank order of certain kinds of shared sentiments in populations. The ability to manipulate oneself or one's program so as to be, or seem to be, in line with these sentiments can, of course, have consequences of great magnitude. Success can lead to being elected prime minister or president or to one's program's being written into law, funded, and staffed. Yet, powerful as they are, popular shared sentiments can nevertheless be based on gross error (the Vietnam War is replete with examples). They can also be transient. The long-range working of social systems is based on many additional structures and functions, some of them far from obvious and not closely linked to issues about which voting is done. It is against these additional structures and functions that programs based on false assumptions come to grief. A good sense for the political winds does not constitute adequate knowledge of those social processes that determine outcomes.

Community and catchment area. It would be helpful to make ever clearer the dissociation of the concept of community from that of catchment area. Our case study illustrates very well that although a board may be drawn from a catchment area it may nevertheless represent neither the catchment area nor any of the numerous communities within it. Realization of this distinction directs attention to the importance of ascertaining in any given area whether the population contains one, several, or no clusters that approximate a chosen operational definition of a community. Open also for ascertainment would be such matters as population mobility, leadership and followership structures, sentiment patterns regarding mental illness care, and so forth. Of particular importance would be detecting qualities such as those termed *community competence* by the sociologist Leonard S. Cotrell.[18] Condensed and paraphrased, these may be listed as follows:

1   Strong sentiments of commitment to work for the benefit of local affairs on the part of community members
2   Ability to define situations clearly
3   Articulateness and capability in communications
4   The capacity to contain conflict and to bring about accommodation
5   Active participation in community affairs
6   Organization for managing relations with the larger society
7   Organization for facilitating collective decision making

Where both the past history of and the ongoing evidence within a population cluster suggest that characteristics such as these are present, then local control and community care of mental illnesses can be expected to have a good chance of success. Where, instead of showing community competence, the population reveals itself to be apathetic, self-disparaging, anomic, and paralyzed, or to be fractured by hostilities, it is certain that these attributes will adversely affect the quality of support systems and services over which the local residents have control and, hence, the lives of those patients "who are returned to their communities."

In some population clusters, the life circumstances of mentally ill people and the management of their care can easily be much worse than in some provincial or state hospitals. It is important to keep in mind that one of the realities that determines outcomes is the fact that there are wide variations across and within catchment areas. Patterns of care giving, therefore, need to be adjusted accordingly. In some areas, the desirable goal may be not community care but, rather, protecting mentally ill individuals from it.

Participant democracy. This realization brings us to the importance of recognizing the potential for conflict between two commonly held sentiments: (1) mentally ill people should have the best possible care, and (2) participant democracy is of paramount importance.[19]

When people are ill, they and their families nearly always wish to have help. Further, they expect that help to be technically correct, honest, dependable, and concerned. They do not want to be exposed to maneuvers that are technically unjustifiable, apathetic, ulterior in motivation, secondary to other considerations, haphazard, misleading, ineffective, or dangerous.

Those who are not ill, and who are not involved with people who are, may also hold to these sentiments, but they may have others pertaining to local autonomy that have a higher priority. In populations with community competence, these can be congruent with quality care. In others, however, the values of local autonomy and participant democracy may produce precisely what ill people and their families do not wish to have: treatment that is technically ignorant, apathetic, ulterior in motivation, secondary to other considerations, haphazard, ineffective, and dangerous.

Blunderings and stumblings in an organization may be tolerable when the concern is with creating a social club, or even a cooperative store. In cases such as the latter, it may be generally agreed that participant democracy is more important than efficient management and profits. The situation may be viewed as a learning experience containing the long-range possibility of progressive improvement, one in which the participants are in a sense learning at their own expense. The situation is different in schools, hospitals, mental health centers, fire departments, airports, and other institutions where malfunctioning can damage lives or kill outright.

It is not, of course, up to the clinical professions to determine the rank order of public values. What we can do, however, is provide facts about alternatives and professional opinions as to what constitutes the best care, given present knowledge, for different kinds of disorders. In this way, we can heighten recognition of the issues and give the public the information it needs to form valid opinions. But we must first achieve greater consensus among ourselves than currently exists.

Governance

The management of any care-giving agency has its share of all the historic, well-known, and largely unsolved problems of human governance. To these are added the individual problems of the particular federal, provincial, or state system of which the agency is a somewhat lowly element. It is also a prisoner of the social structures and sentiment systems in the population it serves.

Nevertheless, there are some issues to be clarified, decisions to be made, and actions to be taken that can render more effective the governance of agencies concerned with mental illnesses. The following seem to me to be important, frequently overlooked, and remediable.

Rewards. The way rewards operate in agencies is in grave need of scrutiny and revision. If an agency is to be successful in fulfilling its assigned goals, it is essential for the members to find that working toward those goals is rewarding. One cannot have an effective army if the soldiers discover it serves them better to run away than to fight.

A truism is a statement that is so obviously true as not to require discussion. My statement above is therefore not a truism because although obviously true, it does require discussion. This is because few policymakers, planners, or administrators appear to accept it, or at least to take it seriously.

Rapid social change and social disintegration have made increasingly common a situation in which the reward system of an organization fails to discriminate between good and bad role performance. As a result, members of the organization seek gratification in other ways, particularly through games of seeking advantage, rather than in the work itself. These games evolve various rules such as "let there be no meritocracy," and are played something like chess with pieces called "seniority," "rights," "influence," "intimidation," "deception," "charm," and "codswallop." The piece called "excellence in role performance" is apt to be little used because it does not help to win games.

Schemes for introducing clinical audit and quality assurance have a potential for bringing goals and motivations into better adjustment with one another, but if they emphasize only the detection of error, they may increase threat and fear of punishment, and thereby generate defenses rather than better work. There is much evidence to suggest that individuals, animal and human, do not give their best in an environment that is mainly threatening. Consequently, agencies that operate with anxiety as their chief motivational force run badly, a tendency which is fostered by the legal adversary approach to correcting organizational defects.

Agencies that run well consist of people playing roles that gratify a plurality of the essential striving sentiments mentioned in Chapter 10. This requires the recognition of willingness and interest and the fostering of urges toward competence, toward helping people, toward being a part of a worthwhile group, and toward seeking recognition and approval for excellence. If monitoring and quality assurance, therefore, are to have beneficial effects on services, they must recognize satisfactory and superior as well as substandard performances.

In sum, for there to be good care of patients, there has to be good care of those who care for them. This rule applies throughout an agency – to people in executive, administrative, and clerical positions as well as to those who have direct contact with patients, and to professionals as well as to paraprofessionals and nonprofessionals.

When the public and the media take a punitive attitude toward agencies that are doing the best they can under difficult circumstances, they destroy rather than correct.

Goals and resources. The age-old, and common nonalignment between agency goals and agency resources needs to be reduced. The resources in question include both money and personnel and have been mentioned many times in the course of this book.

One means of reducing this nonalignment is to increase resources, and this, of course, should be a vigorous concern. It is necessary to be cautious, however, about boosting lofty multiple goals, as has happened so often in movements connected with mental illnesses. Lofty multiple goals bring in money, but they also bring additional expectations along with a high risk of failure and reactions of disillusionment that ultimately work harm on mentally ill individuals, thus more than neutralizing the benefits. The lessons of history point to the importance of preventing the kind of wild swings between overexpectation and disillusionment that have occurred in both distant and recent past.

Another approach to reducing the nonalignment of goals and resources is through adapting the goals of agencies to their resources more strictly and explicitly. In a field as vast in potentials as the one we contemplate, this means a strong sense of priorities. Before we consider priorities, however, let us observe that correcting the nonalignment between goals and resources is an issue for the highest levels of policymakers and requires public understanding, aided by the media. Unless realignment occurs, the governance of agencies will continue as it has been and is, namely, under the strain of overextension, makeshift adaptations, staff vacancies, and perduring malfunction.[20]

Priorities. The development of priorities is a major challenge for the clinical professions because it is as difficult as it is essential. Many writers have recognized its crucial importance; some have offered suggestions such as placing serious psychological disabilities at the top and recommending against the expansion of mental health services and involvement in far-reaching social issues. Most, however, then defeat the purpose of their recommendations by offering long, unsorted, comprehensive lists of targets, thereby showing how difficult it is to leave anything out or even to relegate something to a low priority. One can see this in varying degrees in such major works as *Action for Mental Health, More for the Mind, Today's Priorities in Mental Health,* and the report of the President's Commission.[21]

The nature of the problem is such that it is unlikely ever to be solved by any individual, but it might yield to a task force or a succession of task forces. The manner in which DSM III[22] was developed offers a model and, in addition, a set of foundation stones upon which a system of priorities might be built. If a first approximation to a system of priorities could be achieved within the clinical professions, a more broadly based consensus might be sought through a royal commission or a coalition such as the President's Commission.

Some possible bases on which to develop priorities will be taken up later, in the discussion of a frame of reference.

Division of responsibilities. Clarity with regard to priorities would facilitate a rational division of responsibilities within agencies and among agencies, a necessary step if care-giving services are to rise above their present level. It is essential that social workers, nurses, psychologists, and psychiatrists sort out their competing theories and spheres of influence and move toward better cooperation. Of particular importance is establishing more plainly the role of the general practitioner and family physician and their relationships with the above named professionals. As innumerable writers have said over a great many years and as we found in Stirling County, general practitioners not only are a major source of referral but also actually treat a great many people who are mentally ill. Indeed, our research indicates that they see a much larger percentage of the mentally ill persons in a population than does any other kind of professional.

Policymakers, planners, and administrators, as well as professional associations and professional schools, can help in the development of more coordinated and collaborative patient care among the professions by working out role descriptions that indicate not only the exclusive competencies of each discipline but also the competencies that are shared among two or more; it is important that the shared competencies should be recognized as such. Similar clarity should characterize descriptions of the functions of subunits within organizations so that they are not encouraged by the obscurity of their charges to set upon each other in savage competition.

Interagency cooperation is generally even more troublesome than intraagency cooperation. Any real change in relations between agencies will require drastic alterations in the shared sentiments within the civil service and also within the professions. One influence of importance could be mobilized if administrators were to act so as to make cooperation rewarding. As things are, despite universal praise of cooperation, there is almost no encouragement for carrying it out. For some years, I have made it a practice to ask administrators at all levels in hospitals, outpatient services, social agencies, and other related types of institutions the following question: "When was the last time you promoted someone for interagency cooperation?" The answer is almost always a surprised look, an awkward silence, and then some version of "If I am honest, I'll have to say 'never.'"

The question of a rational division of responsibility for work with mentally ill people brings us to the question of local versus centralized control. What has been said previously, in the discussion of communityism, about great variability in social processes and community competence points to the impossibility of developing any plan that will work well along the whole range of common circumstances.

The dilemma is that both centralized bureaucratic control and local autonomy have enormous capacities for bad performance, as well as some modest potentials for good performance. Resolution of the dilemma is relatively easy if the superordinate value attached to local autonomy is made clear, as discussed earlier in this chapter in regard to participant democracy. One must be prepared in that case, however, to find that in some populations no care is given or, worse, that extraordinarily cruel treatment is provided. But full commitment to centralized control would not necessarily be better. The story of abuses in provincial and state hospitals indicates what can happen when one moves too far in that direction.

If the well-being of mentally ill individuals is accepted as the top priority, then policy regarding the locus of control must incorporate checks and balances and be flexible enough to permit adaption to the variety of social conditions and varying degrees of social integration and disintegration that actually occur in contemporary Western societies. Although foundations for these checks and balances do exist in our political traditions, efforts to establish such a policy are at a severe disadvantage because of the prevalence of communityism and the current disposition toward polarities in political thinking. Such efforts are also complicated by the issue of lay versus professional control and by the fact that long-range principles are often weak in comparison to short-range expediency (which frequently involves personal and political interests).

Patient care as a top priority, therefore, has a tough road ahead. It is surrounded and permeated by issues that are complex and technical but that are also emotional and lend themselves to covert manipulation. Fortunately, the idea of patient care as a top priority is simple and easily understood and can serve well as a guide in the governance of caregiving agencies. What is required is a generally accepted ethic that gives it clear identification as a top priority and that protects it against erosion by "other considerations."

Whether a given mental illness service should have a board and whether that board should be advisory or have executive powers are questions that illustrate the need for flexible policies that take into account the societal characteristics of the area served. The evidence from our case study is that the particular Board studied was never in a position to "direct" the Centre. We cannot rule out the probability that other boards in other contexts could do much better in this regard. It is equally probable, however, that many would do much worse.

What is appropriate, it seems to me, is to foster boards wherever and whenever they will have a constructive influence on patient care, but to have a means for detecting malfunctions that can adversely affect patients. History has shown over and over again that the task of overseeing cannot be safely left entirely to local groups. Well-defined criteria regarding the work of a board would help and could be made to vary selectively from place to place. Minimal standards might include such requirements as ability to keep all seats on the board filled, adequate frequency of attendance at meetings, sufficient supply of people willing and able to assume offices, and stability of membership. Without meeting these requirements, a board has little chance of being a constructive influence in the care of mentally ill people.

Of equal importance is the specification of tasks the board expects to perform. If its function is to be advisory, both the scope and the limitations of the advice expected of it should be made explicit. When advice is to be given, and to whom, should also be stated. If a board's duties are to be directive, the tasks should be explicitly described in such a way as to make it evident to all concerned when they are being accomplished and when not. In particular, the division of responsibility among the board, the central administration, and the staff should be clear to all of them, as well as to those engaged in relevant activities such as peer review and clinical audit. Short-term, renewable contracts between central administration and the board might be one way to achieve both specificity and flexibility. This would be in keeping with the Joint Commission's suggestion that grants to areas should be based on merit.[23]

Crises. Inasmuch as crises are a recurrent pattern in human society, particularly in periods and areas of social disintegration, preparedness for them should be incorporated in the policy of all agencies responsible for the care of mentally ill persons. Guidelines regarding what to do and what not to do should be well thought out in advance and known to all members of the organization, on the model of fire and lifeboat drills. The possibility for this is facilitated by the fact, shown in sociological studies, that many if not most local social crises run very similar courses.

In my view, there is only one position appropriate for a care-giving agency, in a crisis in the area it serves, and that is neutrality. The potential in a crisis for long-lasting destruction of health and well-being outweighs the importance of the issues, however appealing one or the other side may appear at the time. The issues, it often turns out, are more excuses than reasons and frequently have little to do with the course and outcome of the crisis.

Agency neutrality is also a favorable position from which to offer at some point good offices for cooling tensions and finding workable methods for reaching fair-minded solutions. Such a role is especially appropriate for a clinic that deals with mental and emotional problems and is dedicated to the public good.

General problems. Overall, the governance of agencies suffers because the public is insufficiently informed about the processes at work and about many of the issues with which it has to deal, such as those illustrated in our case study. This is a difficult problem to resolve because neither the public nor the media have much inclination toward understanding such complex and somewhat recondite issues. What the public receives in services, therefore, is the product of its common sense mixed with heavy doses of the product of its apathies and its misguided simplistic opinions.

If those who are part of the governing process in care-giving agencies are to have patient care as the first priority, the public will have to be more concerned about the ethics of task accomplishment, not just indignant about "tax payers' money". Equally important, the priority accorded patient care must be written into the goals and searched for in every examination of outcomes. Perhaps each subunit of an agency – clinical teams, committees, and boards – should meet at regular intervals so the members can ask each other the following questions: Are we moving off our patient care target? Are we reenacting without knowing it one or more of the age-old task-defeating patterns? Are we embracing a fad? Are we keeping things in balance? Are we really thinking first about the ill people we serve?

Frame of reference

The consequences of not having an adequate, generally accepted frame of reference for dealing with mental illnesses have appeared in almost every aspect of our case study and in the greater part of the historical and contemporary literature reviewed. Because of the absence of what the Joint Commission called "bench marks and boundary lines,"[24] uncertainty and conflict have repeatedly arisen over what phenomena are to be considered mental illnesses, over how and by whom they are to be treated, over the distinction between treatment and prevention, and over much else. Those participating in and bemused by these confusions include the people that have mental illnesses and their families; the practicing mental health professionals, referring doctors, clergy, social workers, and public health nurses; the mental health association members; and the policymakers at all levels, from local boards to top officials and legislators and, finally, appropriation makers and budget designers. The situation is similar in medical, public health, and social work schools and in other institutions responsible for training and research. Efforts to think clearly, to organize the gathering and analysis of information, to communicate accurately, and to plan effectively flounder in a wilderness of theories and in an enormous vocabulary of terms that stand for loose, variable, and contradictory meanings.

With DSM III (see note 22), a beginning has been made toward constructing a frame of reference that is scientifically valid, that commands a significant degree of consensus, and that opens the possibility of planning by descriptive diagnosis and outcome rather than by myth. This manual rests on many years of study, consultation, and trial and is supported by or congruent with much other work. One of the important gains is progress in separating terms referring to patterns of behavior that can be directly observed and terms referring to psychodynamic processes that can never be directly verified – no matter how plausible they may seem. This distinction is central in making accurate determinations of patient characteristics and patient responses to care, as well as in research of all kinds, whether directed at causes or treatment and whether laboratory, clinical, or epidemiological in its methods.

Standard terms and a widely accepted scientific system of classification are, of course, only the foundation for a frame of reference. It is to be expected that, with experience in use and with contributions from new research, the system of classification will be altered, and one may hope that such changes will be incremental rather than capricious. While the system of classification is developing, other parts of the frame of reference should also receive attention, especially the question of priorities in care giving.

One step in this direction would be the working out of criteria based on facts derived from clinical investigations, laboratory research, and epidemiology. As innumerable epidemiological studies have shown, different classes (diagnostic categories) of mental illnesses have different rates of *prevalence* in populations. Some are common, some are rare, and many are between these poles. Degree of *disability* is also apt to vary, not only among cases within any one class of disorder but also in terms of averages among different classes of disorders. Data on degrees of disability, however, are much less available than data pertaining to prevalence. It is uncommon in treatment records for degree and duration of disability to be systematically noted. There are, however, no insurmountable obstacles to the creation of appropriate procedures for recording disability in terms of both reports on subjective suffering and observable disturbances in social roles and interpersonal relationships.

A third relevant set of facts consists of those derived from clinical studies of *treatability* – that is, the degree to which therapies are effective in relieving disabilities among the different classes of disorders. A considerable amount of information about the efficacy of medications has already been gathered, and it grows yearly. Data regarding various forms of psychotherapy are considerably less trustworthy, a situation that could be improved to some extent by more systematic attention to changes in every patient's condition before, during, and after treatment.

Finally, it may be suggested that the dimensions of prevalence, disability, and treatability could be combined, possibly by means of some system of weights. The psychoses would doubtless emerge in a position of high priority because they are in a large measure both disabling and treatable. Affective disorders, when severely disabling or at risk for suicide, might also have high priority. The very mildly impairing anxiety and depressive disorders (called psychoneuroses before DSM III), pose a special problem. Their great prevalence argues for high priority, but their mildness (which is part of their definition) would suggest low priority. Their treatability involves many complex issues, among them the question of when medication is appropriate and when psychological forms of treatment are to be preferred. Perhaps under most circumstances and for most people, both are desirable. Questions such as these, however, are for research to answer. In the meantime, it is desirable to protect mental illness services from being so overwhelmed with demands for the care of mild chronic affective disturbances that they are unable to give adequate attention to severely disabling types of illnesses that are nevertheless treatable. It may be good policy, therefore, to have alternate systems for care giving such as general practitioners or specialized psychological and social work services, as have evolved for the mentally retarded. Personality disorders present a still more difficult problem because they are so difficult to treat successfully and yet fairly common and often disabling.

That something has to be done for patients with personality disorders is without question, but there is little, if any, evidence at present to justify allocating them to medical (including psychiatric) services.

My intention here is not to go so far as to develop a set of priorities but rather to suggest a direction and to illustrate how data concerning prevalence, disability, and treatability could be combined with data on such additional matters as costs, efficiency, and available resources in money and personnel. What I visualize is that the search for and assembly of data on differential prevalence rates, degrees of disability, and expectable results from treatments would substantially help in the formation of priorities for care and provide guidance for their interpretation on a case-by-case basis. In this way it should be possible to ensure that treatable conditions are treated, particularly those that are disabling and common; and that persons with severe, chronic disturbances that respond little to treatment nevertheless receive such help as would serve to moderate their suffering and the difficulties faced by their families and others around them.[25]

The approach to priorities that has just been suggested does not follow the President's Commission in speaking of priority groups such as children, the elderly, minorities, and others who are socially and economically deprived.[26] These are important groups, of course, some having very high prevalence rates, and they are deprived of adequate services. To focus on them, however, without giving equally prominent attention to discrimination among disorder types is to engage once more in lump thinking and lopsided programming. The concept of *target populations* should be joined to a concept of *target disorders*. To do otherwise is to run the risk of overservicing some groups in a wasteful Lord Ronald fashion while underservicing others. People with serious, common, and treatable illnesses must be reached, whomever or wherever they are.

In addition to supplying the mental illness field with useful consensual categories and establishing criteria for constructing priorities, a further component in a frame of reference would be general agreement as to where the field's *outer boundaries* are. It has been pointed out a number of times in the course of this book that clinicians who deal with mental illnesses often believe that their observations and theories are applicable to every endeavor in which human beings engage: art, philosophy, politics, religion, and science. This belief can be criticized as a foolish and mischievous assumption of omniscience. It contains, however, a modicum of truth inasmuch as people who seek basic knowledge are generally able to find wide use for it. One may add, and still not overclaim, that the study of disordered mentation, emotions, and behavior is one among a number of large windows through which observations can be made, observations that, when joined with those from other windows, help to build a more adequate comprehension of human behavior and its motivations. In this sense, the statements of Meyer and Rennie quoted in Chapter 2, are, I believe, justifiable. But the potential connection of mental illness studies with many profound human issues should not be allowed to become a weak spot in the intellectual structure of the field. It should not be an excuse for permitting the boundary to balloon out and burst scattering fragments in every direction. Neither training in psychiatry nor skill in the diagnosis and treatment of mental illnesses necessarily confers wisdom regarding other aspects of human affairs. Speculation has its place, but it is necessary always to be alert to the risks inherent in the human desire to believe in wondrous stories; the line between intuitive conviction and delusion is thin and permeable. As in medicine generally, policies and practices aimed at the care of mental illnesses should rest on the best available knowledge. To achieve this, however, those of us in the mental illness field must have a strong appreciation of the field's boundaries and of the difference between speculation and reasonably well-established fact. Otherwise, we will wander over an infinite terrain, not knowing whether we are helping or harming until on some far mountain pass we run out of resources.

These considerations are particularly urgent in relation to prevention. People use the claim of preventing mental illnesses as justification for an extremely wide variety of activities. In some instances, belief in the claim has been sincere, but in others it has been more or less a subterfuge to strengthen support for programs that might not otherwise have been supported. When one converts the notion of prevention into the notion of promoting mental health, one invites truly infinite expansion. There is hardly any project concerned with human betterment that cannot be justified under such a heading. Because very little is known about how to prevent most mental illnesses, efforts aimed at prevention mean that resources are deflected from real help for really ill persons to all kinds of diffuse projects. There is also the risk that a field so wide open exposes a clinic to destructive clashing with other agencies and programs that see their interests threatened and their territory invaded. In many ways, mental health efforts are bad for mental illness care.

Both primary and secondary prevention need to be carefully reassessed and their knowledge base defined. Against that background, it might be possible to work toward a consensus about where the margins of caring for mental illnesses lie and where other kinds of major humane endeavors begin – endeavors that should be encouraged and given cooperation but that should not be funded out of budgets for mental illness care. These include public health, welfare services, education, recreation, and other activities that can be, and I think should be, justified in their own right.

It might seem that these remarks indicate a desire to expel primary and secondary prevention from the mental illness field, yet such is not my intention. Prevention should be a major target, but for most types of mental illnesses it should be a research target. The exceptions are those mental disorders that have a known and preventable cause, such as paresis, the psychosis of pellagra, mental retardation secondary to fetal rubella, and brain damage at birth.

The difference between the desire for something and ability to attain is a distinction that is often lost from sight under waves of popular feeling. Pressure to act easily tempts professionals as well as public figures to give the appearance of knowing what is still uncertain and to seem to be engaged in doing what they do not in actuality know how to do. When resources are scarce, it is essential that those resources be guarded from such waste.

Utilization of science

A theme that has evolved in the course of this study is the underutilization of science in coping with mental illnesses. It was evident in microcosm at the Bristol Mental Health Centre in the inability of the staff to conduct research and in the inability of staff, Board, and the provincial Mental Health Administration to utilize the research that was being done in Stirling County on mental illnesses and the social environment.

Part of the difficulty undoubtedly lay in the Stirling County Study's own failure to do an adequate job of communication. In retrospect, it appears certain that we could have done far better in the way we packaged information for staff, Board, and Administration. I doubt, however, that this would have made much difference because no matter how we wrapped our product we would still have been offering it to people who, for a multitude of reasons, had different orientations than ours and too many other things on their minds to be much interested in what was in our package. Most of our concerns were long range, whereas most of theirs were immediate.

In the macrocosm of North America, the picture has been similar. Despite the research that has been done, and despite the unprecedented sums of money that have been spent during the last three decades, there is still something oddly disconnected about the relationship of research to the rest of the mental illness field. It is as if policymakers, planners, administrators, and practitioners consider research to be something apart and unto itself and not a component of their world.

Although the authors of *Action for Mental Health*,[27] published in 1961, give research considerable space and emphasis, both their review of research already done and their recommendations for the future omit almost entirely two areas that are of highest relevance to their principal goal – "services to mentally troubled people" in "their community." The omitted research areas are (1) investigation of the numbers and kinds of mentally troubled people who are to receive these services and (2) the structure and functioning of the communities that are to have demands made on them to support the services. The word *epidemiology* is not in the index of *Action for Mental Health*. The orientation of the authors, however, is reflected in the following statement.

It is commonly stated, on the basis of certain surveys, that one in ten people is mentally ill. This refers to mental illness, major and minor, and includes much mental illness that is not recognized and treated as such. When the number of mentally ill is limited to those coming to professional attention with symptoms disruptive enough to result in diagnosis and hospitalization . . . the ratio is perhaps about one in 100.[28]

(The reader will recall that ten years and five years before this Bremer and Essen-Moeller, respectively, had reported rates of over 20 percent for clinically definable mental illnesses in their studies. See Chapter 2.)

Although this and other statements do not make evident the authors' definition of mental illness or whether, when they speak of service, they are thinking in terms of 10 percent of 1 percent, the book as a whole does indicate that the weight of their concern is with "major mental illness."

More for the Mind, which appeared in Canada in 1963, did not touch at all on the topic of research. Some of the consequences in the form of inappropriate planning that can occur as a result of such lack of concern were described by Martin et al. in 1976.[29]

The report of the President's Commission, published seventeen years after *Action for Mental Health,* again attaches great importance to research, even though "our national capacity has undergone severe erosion" in the interim. These authors also mention the 10-percent figure but regard it as minimal and suggest that 15 percent may be more realistic. The relevance of epidemiology is recognized and its development strongly recommended. But the importance and relevance of research into the structure and functioning of communities together with transcommunity social and economic systems does not emerge as very important in the report except insofar as these can be classified as support systems. These questions seem to rest more or less where they were when the Joint Commission passed them by, and the report is still pervaded by individualism and communityism.[30]

The report places appropriate emphasis on the lack of research manpower but does not appear to consider that past failures to take seriously or utilize research results may have been significant factors in discouraging people from entering research. The problem is formidable with great obstacles arrayed against anyone who would try to resolve it. Nevertheless, it is possible to suggest the following points in regard to utilizing science.

Research on the underutilization of scientific research. The question of why there are so many blind spots that interfere with utilizing scientific information in policymaking, planning, and administration in the mental illness field is one which itself deserves scientific research. The underutilization is almost certainly due in part to the state of the field. Given the evident welter of contradictions and confusions, and the lack of an agreed-upon frame of reference, policymakers, planners and administrators have good reason to be cautious about what are offered to them as scientific findings. It is also apparent that research workers are often not very adept in presenting their results in a way that policymakers can understand and appreciate.

These difficulties, the overcoming of which might be considered the responsibility of the researchers, are not, however, sufficient to explain nonutilization. Something more forceful is at work.[31] The distaste for science and the susceptibility to fads to be discussed below are likely influences, and their effects on policy need to be better understood. The problem, however, is not only the individual policymaker's personal sentiments but also the question of how new information is apt to affect his position. Does it threaten a previously established social as well as psychological equilibrium? Does it demand that he engage in activities for which he has neither the knowledge nor the skills? Does he see research as the enemy of a controllable status quo and the harbinger of unwelcome uncertainties? Does he think it threatens him with obsolescence?

It can also be suspected that important components of the problems lie in the kinds of education, training and experience the policymakers, planners, and administrators have in their backgrounds. Do they, like many lawyers and some doctors, arrive in their roles without acquiring an adequate grasp of what the scientific process is and of how to sift and utilize its results? Some policymakers have been known to complain that scientists present them with too many "ifs and buts" and "one hands and other hands," and no doubt this is troublesome. At the same time, it is important for them to appreciate that true statements may be subtle, complex, and relative because such is the nature of the phenomena they describe. Marc Lalonde is perhaps right when he says that "messages designed to influence the public must be loud, clear and unequivocal,"[32] but it is important for him and other men and women in public life to realize that in human affairs such statements are often also wrong.

How do the structures and systems of sentiment in agencies and policy-forming groups affect the kinds of information that are accepted or rejected, and in what ways is information that is accepted utilized? What constraints are put upon the individual that render his survival in his role dependent upon responsiveness to conventional wisdom and popular ideas, regardless of evidence about their validity? Is the resistance to new scientific information simply a particular expression of the much more widely observed tendency of societies to resist social innovations unless they appear capable of meeting some strongly felt immediate need? Do we understand adequately the momentum-like phonomenon mentioned in the earlier discussion of communityism in the mental health center movement? (The reader will recall that after a certain point it became virtually impossible for the proponents to turn away from unrealistic emphasis on the community.) Is a point of no return apt to be characteristic of policy formation and is it possible to find ways to make policy formation more flexible and responsive to new information?

There is much knowledge now available about the functioning of human organizations, and there are also many relevant research methods that could be much more effectively utilized than they have been in those organizations concerned with mental illnesses.

Fear of science. The fact that many people are afraid of science is a problem that deserves fuller recognition. In the present day of nuclear weapons, industrial pollution, and changes in the way of life brought about by technology, it is very likely that apprehension and mistrust attach to every brand of science. There can be little doubt, however, that those sciences that probe the mind are especially vulnerable. People dislike the idea of having their inner psychological workings laid bare, and they are unhappy with the thought that scientists might actually succeed in doing so. Nearly everyone fears being shown that the self is nothing but a mass of psychological predispositions and predictable responses; the individual fears being turned from a "me" into a machine. In these terms, science seems to diminish personal worth and moral purpose to the zero point and to arouse fearful images of mind-controlling bureaucratic systems. A focus on mental illness adds to this all the emotional turbulence outlined previously as barrier two.

Not the least important aspect of the fear of science as applied to mental illnesses is the fact that many psychiatrists, psychologists, and other professionals must be numbered among those who share this feeling. Almost every clinician wishes to have the dignity and prestige of being regarded as scientific, but many find the actual mode of thought to be tedious, uncongenial, or disturbing. The latter can be seen, for instance, in much of the plainly emotional antagonism some people display toward systems of nosology, where the human being is pictured as vanishing in a heap of meaningless labels.[33]

The problem deserves not only research aimed at better understanding but also more discussion of such questions as the following: To what extent are the antagonisms based on misunderstandings of science and to what extent are they well justified? Is it important to introduce humanistic values when science is applied to policy formation and planning? If so, what are the best procedures for accomplishing this?

At the present time, it can no longer be assumed as an article of faith that all kinds of scientific inquiry are intrinsically good, in either the short or the long run. It is, however, appropriate to maintain that any constraints on investigation should be rational and based on the best understanding possible of both the scientific and the nonscientific considerations involved.

Susceptibility to fads. As mentioned earlier in this chapter, the mental illness field has always been, and continues to be, afflicted with unsubstantiated beliefs, mistaken assumptions, and mischievous half-truths. The word *fad* might be employed except that it carries unfortunate connotations of triviality, such as in matters of dress or hairstyle. The fads in ideas are often far from trivial; they have a potential for turning malignant and spreading like forest fires, as was evident in Nazi Germany. There can be little doubt, to give a medical illustration, that the once fashionable notion of bleeding the sick led to innumerable deaths; used during the period called the Enlightenment, it probably killed more mentally ill people than were burned in previous centuries for witchcraft. The total history of treatment for mental illnesses is a long and at times exceedingly cruel one, and its fads appear on occasion to be the expression of surges of conscious and unconscious hatred of insane persons.

Dealing with fads, however, is difficult, partly because there are so many false and dubious notions that come and go, partly because they are hard to disprove, and partly because while they last they involve formidable amounts of money and political power. They attract supporters, including professionals in the mental illness field, who develop one or another kind of vested interest in keeping them going as long as possible. These persons, both singly and in groups, attack with great vigor those who challenge and seek to test for evidence.

It cannot be claimed that science provides sure, effective remedies, but it can be claimed that science has some strengths and offers some resources that could be used more than they are to monitor validity and to defend the well-being of mentally ill persons. It is also important that research be focussed on what it is that generates widely shared false beliefs and on how to prevent wasteful or malignant outcomes. The need for developing public and legal opinion that would be more adequately informed and more supportive of efforts to ascertain validity is apparent.

Society and the care of mental illnesses. The effect of society on the care of mental illnesses is a topic about which information has begun to accumulate. Some years ago, Hollingshead and Redlich[34] demonstrated that socioeconomic class level is associated with type of treatment, and there have also appeared numbers of other indications of a similar sort in the literature. The present book, too, has pointed to different aspects of social structure and social process that shape and limit the functioning of caregiving programs.

This is a type of research that deserves to be pushed much further than it has been, particularly with regard to the processes of governance. I think it likely that the sociological and psychological factors at work in medical and other care-giving agencies are different in important ways from those in the higher echelons of government and in profit-making organizations. This means that at least some of what is taught as "policy" and "management science" in schools of government and business administration is probably wrong when applied to clinical and helping services, particularly in regard to motivations, patterns of reward, and other potentials for improving performance.

The reverse relationship, the effect of programs for the care of mental illnesses on society, is a major blank in our understanding. Do different kinds of programs interact differently with the subsystems of the society they touch? Are there ramifying, unrecognized effects? Do some programs more than others inspire counterreactions, or cause people to turn away? Do some kinds of programs impose severe burdens on, or threaten, those who are well? Is it possible that the decline of the various major movements in the mental illness field are in part due to negative societal reactions against burdens imposed by these care-giving subsystems? And are some of the subsystems more successful than others in avoiding counterreactions?

Many different patterns of care are now being tried in various places, and there is, consequently, opportunity to trace and compare their effects, if any, on families, religious and recreational groups, employers, unions, social services, local and central governments, and other networks, and also on communities. There is opportunity to see to what extent the various program goals are harmonious or at variance with the shared sentiments characteristic of the populations affected.

Society and mental illnesses. There is almost no systematic knowledge regarding the effect of mental illnesses on society. The fact that the vast bulk of efforts in social psychiatry has been toward elucidating how social factors affect mental illnesses reflects an outstanding bias in the way we look at human problems. Clinicians interested in research have concentrated on elucidating causes and developing therapies. Social scientists have, to a very large extent, focused on mental illnesses as the product of social perceptions and practices. Yet the converse questions are as important as any of these, and have been ever since science began to concern itself with mental illnesses. Recognition of the fact that there is such a thing as stigma automatically prompts the question of why it exists, but this question has rarely been pursued except in speculative terms.

The realization that the prevalence rates for all kinds of mental illnesses considered together range from 15 to 25 percent puts the question in a new light and increases its urgency. This is a very large number of people whose disabilities must be having far-reaching effects on how social systems of all kinds function. The problem is therefore not only psychological, psychiatric, medical, and social in nature but also one that affects economics, human relations, institutional management, and government.

The above remarks are not a reassertion of the theory-based claim sometimes made by psychoanalysts that "everyone needs treatment." They are the logical result of counting the number of people impaired because of clinically definable disorders.

Prevention. The desirability of designating prevention as primarily a research problem was mentioned in the section on the frame of reference. It is only necessary, therefore, to add a few supplemental remarks.

Because the prevention of mental illnesses would be an overwhelmingly important activity if it were feasible, research on prevention deserves an exceedingly high priority in national, provincial, and state policies. It must be anticipated that studies will be long and costly due to the time dimensions and multiple factors involved and to the difficulties of measuring outcomes. We are fortunate, however, in already having a fairly cogent body of theory on which manageable projects can be based. Many of these might be similar to the prevention efforts of the past, but they could be selected for their susceptibility to monitoring and the measurement of results.

My emphasis on separating prevention research from services applies to projects, but not to personnel. I wish to underline inquiry as a separate objective, as well as independence of funding, but not physical and organizational detachment. Although some kinds of projects might, indeed, be completely independent, others would be better if located in mental health centers or in the mental illness units of health centers. Further, the service personnel could participate part-time in the research, thus ensuring an interchange of clinical and research ideas. Separation of prevention research from service should be maintained only to the extent necessary to ensure that spreading into diffuse and measureless projects does not occur and that scientific standards are maintained.

Orientation of scientific research. Implicit in all the preceding points is the belief that research should be problem oriented rather than discipline oriented. This is a consequence of the fact that most of the important questions, whether heuristic or applied, have too many components to be answerable through the knowledge and skill of any one discipline alone. Significant progress depends on recognizing this and organizing work accordingly.

Such problem-oriented organization of work could result in improved relationships among all disciplines in the mental illness field. The act of working jointly and reciprocally on target questions could do much to give each discipline a better perspective on itself and on others in relation to available knowledge, available resources, and the frontier of unsolved problems. It could also facilitate advance toward a strategy proposed by Lalonde: "an ongoing dialogue between health planners and the research community on the priorities for mission-oriented health research while preserving for the research community the setting of priorities in basic research."[35]

My suggestion that there is a need for more and different kinds of research does not disregard numerous inherent difficulties in the questions discussed and does not maintain that a big enough push in research would solve everything. My desire is rather to see a better job done of finding the right place for research within the total care-giving and educational complex. As *The Lancet* has said, "such a mix cannot be found by guesswork or intuition derived from clinical experience. It requires a scientific approach."[36]

Concluding note

The problems with which the phenomena of mental illnesses confront mankind are formidable. It is because they are so formidable that they are still with us after so many years and so much effort. No cultural group and no period in history, so far as we know, has succeeded in eliminating them. Thus it is that we find our hopes of 1950 thrust back upon us by the experiences of trying to fulfill them.

Yet these are not reasons for giving up. It is still possible to think that the ethical frame and goals to which the Bristol Mental Health Centre was dedicated were right. The fact that we did not achieve our ideal does not vitiate the possibility of creating marked advances in mental illness care. Understanding why things go wrong helps us to see how to make them go more advantageously. We now have, as a result of effort and trials, a more detailed map – even if it is still incomplete – than we had before. The fact that it tells us that the terrain is far more complicated and rugged than we had thought is an opportunity to improve our approach. It provides guidance for creating more adequate conceptual tools, more competent service organizations, more effective research, and more appropriate educational backups.

Perhaps most of all, it points to the importance of detecting unfounded beliefs and pulling them out, roots and all. This is because, as we have seen, policies in mental illness care, like other policies, are determined by opinions, whereas outcomes are determined by realities. The challenge is to find ways and means for bringing opinions and realities closer together.

Appendix A

Excerpts from the Bristol Centre's
Memorandum of Association, Bylaws, and
Policies and Regulations

The *Memorandum of Association* states the Board's objectives to be as follows:

a   To maintain and operate a mental health clinic at Bristol, to furnish mental health services to residents of the Counties of Kingston, Stirling, and Harwich;
b   To provide, upon request from the proper authorities, a mental health service for patients in any of the residential institutions in these areas regardless of the home residence of the patients;
c   To provide a consultation service in respect to mental health for the physicians practising in the area;
d   To provide educational material and disseminate information concerning mental health;
e   To accumulate knowledge and analyse information obtained by the Centre as a basis for research into local problems;
f   To provide opportunity for observation, instruction, and research in mental health matters;
g   To do all such other acts and things as are incidental or conducive to or consequential upon the attainment of the foregoing purposes.

The relevant parts of the *Bylaws* state the following:

12   There shall be a Board of Directors composed of sixteen members . . . ;
13   The Directors shall be appointed for a period of two years each provided, however, that the Directors first appointed shall only hold office until the first annual meeting to be held in March 1957;
14   Retiring Directors are eligible for re-election;
15   The Executive Director and all other employees of the Clinic will be appointed by the Board. The Executive Director will be the Secretary to the Board and will attend all meetings, will keep all records except the financial, and will prepare an annual statement of work done for submission to the Board. He will act as advisor to the Board but will be without vote at meetings;
16   The Board will elect its own Chairman at first meeting. No Chairman shall serve in this capacity for more than two consecutive years;
17   A quorum for a Board meeting will be seven members not counting the Secretary;
18   The Board shall meet quarterly: in March, June, September, and December or at any time that a meeting is called at the request of any two members. The March meeting will be termed the Annual Meeting;

19   No employee of the Clinic may at the same time be a member of the Board of Directors;

20   The Executive Director will be the Administrative Officer and will have under his supervision the direction of Clinic activities within any limits imposed by the Board of Directors. He may hire or suspend employees pending approval of such action by the Board.

Powers of directors

1   To take such steps as they think fit to carry into effect any agreement or contract made by or on behalf of the society;

2   To determine who shall be entitled to sign on the society's behalf, bills, notes, receipts, acceptances, endorsements, cheques, releases, contracts, and documents;

3   To make, vary, and appeal rules for the regulation of the business of the society, or of its officers and servants;

36   The society may alter or add to its by-laws at any general meeting of the society and any alteration or addition so made shall be as valid as if originally contained in the by-laws, provided, however, that notice of such intention to alter or amend the by-laws shall be given in the notice calling such general meeting.

The word *society* refers to the parent organization that elected the Centre's Board of Directors. Any resident of the area served by the Centre was eligible for membership on paying an annual fee of one dollar. All this was in conformity with the province's Societies Act, by which the Board became a legal entity. Inasmuch as very few people aside from the Board members joined the society, it was largely fictitious.

The *Policies and Regulations with Regard to Grants-in-Aid to Community Mental Health Boards,* which expressed the Mental Health Administration's views, although they had frequently been stated verbally, were not circulated in writing until 1962. The relevant parts are as follows:

The members of the Board shall be chosen to represent as wide a variety of important and representative groups of the community as possible.

One or more practicing physicians in the Region shall be appointed to the Board.

The Director of the Health Unit shall also be a member.

The Administrator of the Mental Health Services or his representative shall be an ex-officio member of the Board without the privilege of voting.

Other non-voting Board members may be appointed if this is felt desirable.

Functions

The Mental Health Boards shall survey the mental health needs of the Region and shall try to provide as complete a mental health service to it as is possible consistent with its staff and financial resources. Such services include the following:

Service to patients
Service to organizations, agencies, and professional personnel concerned
with mental disorder and mental health
Education
Prevention
Research
Other matters

The policies to be adopted in the organization of these services include the
following:

Service to Patients

Mental health services shall be provided to both adults and children unless otherwise specified.

Patients may be seen in the headquarters established by the Board or in such
other places as may be agreed upon. Home visits may be made if this is felt desirable.

Patients may be accepted on referral by physicians, Health and Welfare agencies, Children's Aid Societies, courts, schools, etc. Self referrals may be accepted
if this is agreed to by the Board.

In providing such services, the Board shall work as closely and co-operatively
as possible with other personnel and facilities interested in caring for the mentally
ill. These include the following:

1. *The local practising physician.*

2. *The Public Health Unit.* A working relationship should be set up with the
Health Unit Director and the Public Health Nurses so that mental health needs of
the Region can be dealt with co-operatively.

3. *The local general hospital.* It should be pointed out that the costs of psychiatric inpatients in general hospitals are payable by the Hospital Insurance Commission on the same basis as are other patients.

4. *The Nova Scotia Hospital.* The role played in relation to patients admitted to
and discharged from the Nova Scotia Hospital shall be worked out in collaboration with the practising physicians in the Region, the Public Health Unit, the Nova
Scotia Hospital, and the Division of Mental Health Services.

To facilitate the carrying out of such a program as may be agreed upon, it is
desirable for the Board to instruct its staff to visit the Nova Scotia Hospital at
reasonable intervals, at least once every three months.

5. *Municipal Mental Hospitals.* The Board shall establish a relationship with
the Municipal Mental Hospital in the Region and with such other Municipal Mental Hospitals as may be agreed upon by the Board and the Mental Health Services.
The services provided to such hospitals shall include the following:

All patients in such Municipal Mental Hospitals shall be examined at least once
a year and reports and recommendations submitted to the Superintendent of the
Hospital and to the Division of Mental Health Services.

Individual patients shall be examined at the Hospital from time to time upon
request of the Mental Health Services and such reports on them shall be submitted
as are requested.

Other or additional services for the Municipal Mental Hospitals shall be provided as may be agreed upon by the Board in collaboration with the Hospital authorities and the Mental Health Services.

Service to organizations, agencies, and professional personnel concerned with mental disorder and mental health

In the preceding sections, interest was centered on the patient himself and on medical personnel and facilities. Here we are concerned with the relationships to be established with other organizations and facilities which deal with, or have an interest in, mental illness and mental health.

No attempt will be made to make a complete list of all such organizations and facilities. The following official and voluntary bodies, among others, have received help from Mental Health Boards:

The Provincial Department of Public Welfare

Municipal Departments of Welfare and their agents

Juvenile Courts

Reformatories

Public Schools and other educational bodies

Family and Welfare Agencies

Children's Aid Societies

The Canadian Mental Health Association

The Canadian Association for Retarded Children

The Canadian Association for Crippled Children and Adults

No definite standards can be written about these relationships, but it is expected that the Board will do what it can to cooperate with some of these or other organizations and facilities. In some cases, these organizations will request examinations of individual patients, such as children being considered for adoption, problem children in schools, persons under the care of the Department of Public Welfare, individuals appearing before the courts, etc. In others, what will be desired are conferences on a regular or irregular basis with professional personnel of the organizations, so that such personnel will be better able to handle their own patients and cases. Or, the requests may be for assistance in other ways.

Special note should be made about services to persons before the courts. It is recommended that the professional staff of the Boards do not take sides in a legal issue, but that any report they make be made available to the judge, the prosecution, and the defence.

Prevention

Prevention in general medicine is traditionally classified into three types. Primary prevention is where the aim is to prevent a disease from occurring at all. Secondary prevention is the attempt to discover and treat a disorder in its early stages so that it does not develop into its full form. Tertiary prevention is simply the proper treatment of a patient with a well developed disorder with an aim of preventing later complications or permanent disabilities.

Secondary and tertiary preventions will automatically take place in any well run program operated by the Board. Primary prevention is more difficult to obtain. This is so for two main reasons. The first is that in many instances we are not sure of the precise cause of the mental disorder we are attempting to cure. The second is that where we do know the cause, and where we think we do, it is frequently very difficult to eradicate.

The Board should give serious thought to all three forms of prevention.

Research

Research into matters pertaining to mental disorder and mental health should be considered one of the important functions of the Board bearing in mind the other programs that have to be carried out.

The Board may apply through the Administrator of Mental Health Services for a Federal-Provincial Grant for research. Such grants are considered in November of each year. Staff who are paid full-time by grants-in-aid cannot be given additional honoraria through such research grants.

Other functions

The Board may undertake such other functions as appear to it desirable.

Administration

The Board shall provide a headquarters for its operations in a suitable location and may arrange for additional facilities at other places if these are needed for adequate coverage of the Region. The location of these facilities shall be decided upon by the Board with the agreement of the Mental Health Services.

Staff

The Board is responsible for the recruitment, hiring, work, discipline, and discharge of the staff. All staff members are employees of the Board and are responsible to the Board. They are not employees of the Provincial Government.

Program

The Board shall plan the overall program and ensure that the different functions are carried out in reasonable proportions and that the whole Region is covered as adequately as possible. It shall see to it that the time of the staff is properly budgeted to this end.

The program so prepared by the Board shall be approved by the Mental Health Services unless it contravenes the generality of the preceding clauses.

The Mental Health Services may inquire at any time into the nature of the program going on and may require that the agreed upon functions be carried out.

Records and reports

The Board shall have adequate records kept of the services rendered to patients, of the staff activities, of the financial operations, and of the work of the Centre generally. The nature of these records will be determined by the Administrator of Mental Health Services in collaboration with the Centres.

The financial records shall be subject to provincial and federal audit.

A full report of the program carried out and a complete financial statement shall be prepared and copies sent to the Mental Health Services at the end of each year.

Grants-in-aid

Mental Health Boards which are approved and meet the standards laid down in previous sections are eligible to receive grants-in-aid from the Province. These grants will reimburse the Board for certain expenditures.

Nothing herein shall prevent a Board from providing additional salaries, leave with pay, honoraria or other such extra benefits as it may wish to provide for its staff; but a Board shall not be reimbursed by grants-in-aid for such extra benefits over and above those provided for under Civil Service schedules of pay and regulations.

Appendix B

Memorandum of November 24, 1955

The Bristol Mental Health Centre has been the only psychiatric service in Western Nova Scotia during the past five years. While it has served mainly Stirling County during this time, it has also given some service to both Harwich and Kingston Counties.

During the past four years the Centre has carried out a major service function in Stirling County. About 75 percent of the Centre Staff's time, over the past four years, has been devoted to helping more than 500 individuals to deal with their emotional problems. The Centre's work with these patients has varied from diagnostic and consultative work, through short term psychotherapy to a few cases of fairly prolonged intensive psychotherapy. The Centre has done both outpatient and inpatient E.C.T. treatment at the Bristol General Hospital and has in the last year made more general use of such tranquilizing drugs as Rauwolfia and Chlorpromazine. The remainder of the staff's time has been divided between community activity and research. Under the rubric of community activity we would include such tasks as rehabilitation of patients returning from mental institutions, acting in a consultative and education role with such community agencies as the clergy and the Social Welfare workers, and working along with the local Mental Health Association. Research activities in the past include among other things studies of the incidence of psychological symptoms in the population which we serve and intensive studies of the mode of transmission of symptoms within a family group.

This research is part of a larger research programme being carried out in Stirling County by Cornell University, with funds financed through the University; and as such, it is a major contribution to the economic well-being of the area.

The extent of such benefit can be estimated from the fact that the total Cornell Project budget for the last three years has been about $113,000.00 per annum, most of which was spent in Stirling County. Of this amount, $3,000.00 per annum was provided by the Nova Scotia Provincial Government, $30,000.00 by the Federal Government through Dominion Provincial Grants and the majority, about $80,000.00 per year, from prominent American research foundations.

The clinic's purposes

1. To institute a service similar to the one outlined above to a wider area of Western Nova Scotia, specifically Harwich County and the Western part of

240

Kingston County. The Centre plans to open a part-time office in Harwich within the next year.

2. To cooperate fully with all community agencies who wish to use its services.

3. To continue a basic research programme building upon the work already done. This programme will continue to attract research funds to the area.

Why the Centre must be a research organization

The Province of Nova Scotia has been unable to staff its Clinics in other parts of the Province. Bristol has been able to keep a capable psychiatric staff because the opportunity for research is attractive to well qualified psychiatrists. We are convinced that without a research connection, the Bristol Mental Health Centre would be in the same position as many other decentralized clinics such as Harwich, that is, without staff. Thus we feel that the Centre must be a research organization if it is to function at all. From this some might infer that one simply had to pay more per service in rural areas. We do not feel that this is necessarily the case. As the result of past resources, the Centre has a great deal of information on file; this information, collected for research purposes, often enables us to help patients far more quickly than would otherwise be the case. Proposed future researches, such as one projected into the functions of the Centre as an organization in the community or one into reasons why some people with symptoms come to a psychiatric clinic while others do not, will rely almost entirely for data on material which a good clinic would collect routinely in any case. The location of the Centre in Bristol not only makes operation in this sense easier and more profitable because of the vast store of basic material on file, but enables the Centre to use its accumulated prestige with research foundations to obtain further grants. Since these grants would be very difficult to obtain in another location and since the continuation of the basic research programme for an extended period will require such grants, we feel that an efficient psychiatric service for Western Nova Scotia can only be provided through a service and research clinic based at Bristol.

Implications for Centre research policy

Research in such a situation becomes not a privilege accorded to some person to gratify a whim but a basic and integral part of the Centre's functioning – If the research is poorly carried out the Centre may lose its support and fail to continue as a research organization. If our thesis which we have developed above is true, this would also mean its demise as a service organization.

If on the other hand service is not of the best quality, the quality of material for research will suffer, the goodwill of the community will lessen and thus make research harder to do and the clinic will again find itself in difficulties. The task of the administrator must be, therefore, to administer the Centre so that its many tasks can all be carried out efficiently. We believe that for the present, at any rate, the Centre can meet its obligations with the resources which it has budgeted.

Research has in the past, through direct subsidy and by means of the personnel which it has attracted for training, supported the service programme. Our present budget attempts to deal with this unstable situation by converting a larger portion of its total into highly skilled personnel. By so doing, it is felt that the clinic can be self sustaining in the service aspects financially. Similarly, research beyond the minimal basic programme will also have to find outside funds for its existence. They will we hope continue to coexist, mutually financially independent but with great benefit one to the other.

Notes

1. Introduction

1. The President's Commission on Mental Health, Report to the President, Washington, D.C., U.S. Government Printing Office, 1978.

2. M. Beiser, R. Krell, T. Lion, and M. H. Miller, eds., *Today's Priorities in Mental Health – Knowing and Doing*, Miami, Symposia Specialists, 1978.

3. R. Dahrendorf, quoted by F. A. Binks, "Changing the subject," *The Lancet*, July 1, 1978, Vol. II, no. 8079, p. 32.

4. Alexander H. Leighton, *My Name is Legion: Foundations for a Theory of Man in Relation to Culture*, New York, Basic Books, 1959.

5. See, for example, Alexander H. Leighton, and Dorothea C. Leighton, *The Navaho Door*, Cambridge, Mass., Harvard University Press, 1944; Alexander H. Leighton, *The Governing of Men*, Princeton, N.J., Princeton University Press, 1945; Alexander H. Leighton, *Human Relations in a Changing World*, New York, E. P. Dutton, 1949; and Tom T. Sasaki, *Fruitland New Mexico: A Navaho Community in Transition*, Ithaca, N.Y., Cornell University Press, 1961.

2. Barriers to effective mental health care

1. See, for example, P. I. Ahmed and S. C. Plog, *State Mental Hospitals: What Happens When They Close*, New York, Plenum Medical Book Co., 1976; E. L. Bassuk and L. Gerson, "Deinstitutionalization and mental health services," *Scientific American*, vol. 238, no. 2, 1978, pp. 48–53; and S. A. Kirk and M. E. Therrien, "Community mental health myths and fate of former hospitalized patients," *Psychiatry*, vol. 38, August 1975, pp. 209–17.

2. Insufficient appreciation of the heterogeneity of mental illness phenomena has also affected research. In some instances, it has led to rather uncritical leaning on speculations about a unitary concept of mental illness, in others to difficulties in comprehending that different epidemiological studies often focus on different kinds of mental illnesses, and in still others to mistaking instruments developed for the identification of psychoneurosis for instruments designed to identify mental illnesses of every form. For examples of each of these, see L. Srole, T. S. Langner, S. T. Michael, M. K. Opler, and T. A. C. Rennie, *Mental Health in the Metropolis: The Midtown Manhattan Study*, New York, McGraw-Hill, 1962, p. 153; B. P. Dohrenwend, and B. S. Dohrenwend, "The problem of validity in field studies of psychological disorder," *Journal of Abnormal Psychology*, Vol. 70, no. 1, 1965, pp. 52–69; and M. Tousignant, G. Denis, and R. Lachapella, "Some considerations concerning the validity and use of the health opinion survey," *Journal of Health and Social Behavior*, vol. 15, 1974, pp. 241–52.

3. For example, see T. Scheff, *Being Mentally Ill: A Sociological Theory*, Chicago, Aldine, 1966; and M. Siegler, H. Osmond, *Models of Madness, Models of Medicine*, New York, Macmillan, 1974, pp. 65–87.

243

4. Speaking in the third person, Newton said, "It must be allowed that these two Gentlemen differ very much in Philosophy. The one proceeds upon the evidence arising from experiments and phenomena, and stops where such evidence is wanting; the other is taken up with hypotheses, and propounds them, not to be examined by experiments, but to be believed without an examination" (Quoted by Alan E. Shapiro, *Science,* vol. 210, October 24, 1980, p. 417).

5. H. Owens, and J. S. Maxmen, "Mood and affect: A semantic confusion," *American Journal of Psychiatry,* vol. 136, no. 1, 1979, pp. 97–9.

6. A. Meyer, "Progress in Psychiatric Teaching," in Eunice E. Winters, ed., *The Collected Papers of Adolf Meyer,* Baltimore, The Johns Hopkins University Press, 1951, pp. 46–7.

7. T. A. C. Rennie, "Social psychiatry: A definition," *International Journal of Social Psychiatry,* vol. 1, 1955, pp. 5–14. For discussions of some of the problems raised by these ideas, see M. G. Miller and M. B. Schwarm, *Mental Illness and the Problem of Boundaries,* Washington, D. C., Medicine in the Public Interest, 1976; and Nina Ridenour, "A Nucleus but No Boundary," in *Mental Health in the United States – A Fifty Year History* (Chapter 3), Cambridge, Mass., Harvard University Press (for the Commonwealth Fund), 1961, pp. 121–31.

8. H. C. Rumke, "Solved and unsolved Problems in Mental Health: The President's Address," in William Line and M. O. King, eds., *Mental Health and Public Affairs,* Toronto, University of Toronto Press, 1954, p. 149.

9. For example, see A. Kardiner, *The Psychological Frontiers of Society,* New York, Columbia University Press, 1945; A. H. Leighton, *Human Relations in a Changing World,* New York, E. P. Dutton, 1949; A. S. Stouffer, A. A. Lumsdaine, M. H. Lumsdaine, et al., *The American Soldier: Combat and Its Aftermath,* Vol. 2, Princeton University Press, 1949.

10. For example, see P. J. Fink and S. P. Weinstein, "Whatever happened to psychiatry? The deprofessionalization of community mental health centers," *American Journal of Psychiatry,* vol. 136, no. 4A, 1979, pp. 406–9; L. Glass, "Psychiatric disturbances associated with Erhard Seminars Training," *American Journal of Psychiatry,* vol. 134, no. 3, 1977, p. 245; H. Gottesfeld, *The Critical Issues of Community Mental Health,* New York, Behavioral Publications, 1972; A. H. Leighton, "Research directions in psychiatric epidemiology," *Psychological Medicine,* vol. 9, 1979, pp. 235–47; E. D. Rosen, *Psychobable,* Atheneum, New York, 1975; D. L. Rosenhan, "On being sane in insane places," *Science,* vol. 179, 1973, pp. 250–8.

11. A. Lewis, "Phillipe Pinel and the English," *The State of Psychiatry,* New York, Science House (originally published by Routledge and Kegan Paul, London), 1967, pp. 9–10.

12. J. Bremer, "A social psychiatric investigation of a small community in northern Norway," *Acta Psychiatrica et Neurologica Scandinavica* Supplementum, vol. 62, 1951, p. 85.

13. E. Essen-Moeller, "Individual traits and morbidity in a Swedish rural population," *Acta Psychiatrica et Neurologica Scandinavica* Supplementum, vol. 100, 1956, pp. 154–5.

14. For example, see D. C. Leighton, J. S. Harding, D. B. Macklin, A. M. Macmillan, and A. H. Leighton, *The Character of Danger: Psychiatric Symptoms in Selected Communities,* New York, Basic Books, 1963, p. 142; D. C. Leighton, J. S. Harding, D. B. Macklin, C. C. Hughes, and A. H. Leighton, "Psychiatric findings of the Stirling County study," *American Journal of Psychiatry,* vol. 119, no. 11, 1963, pp. 1021–6.

15. Srole et al., *Mental Health in the Metropolis,* p. 138.

16. M. Kramer, E. S. Pollack, R. Redick, and B. Z. Locke, *Mental Disorders – Suicide,* Cambridge, Mass., Harvard University Press, 1966, p. 75.

17. The Diagnostic and Statistical Manual (DSM-I, 1952) of the American Psychiatric Association, for example, was exceedingly comprehensive. The Stirling County Study pointed out that if one adhered to the criteria of the manual, the result would be a prevalence rate of 57% rather than 20%. See J. M. Murphy, "Continuities in community-based psychiatric epidemiology," *Archives of General Psychiatry,* vol. 37, 1980, pp. 1215–23.

18. For example, see R. B. Caplan, *Psychiatry and the Community in Nineteenth-Century America,* New York, Basic Books, 1969; G. N. Grob, *Mental Institutions in America: Social Policy to 1875,* New York, The Free Press, 1973; J. C. Perry, "Four Twentieth-Century Themes in Community Mental Health Programs," in B. H. Kaplan, R. N. Wilson, and A. H. Leighton, eds., *Further Exploration in Social Psychiatry,* New York, Basic Books, 1976.

19. J. A. Talbott, "Care of the chronically mentally ill – still a national disgrace. Editorial," *American Journal of Psychiatry,* vol. 136, no. 5, 1979, pp. 688–9. See also The President's Commission on Mental Health, *Report to the President,* Washington, D.C., U.S. Government Printing Office, 1978, pp. 22–6.

20. Grob, *Mental Institutions in America;* N. Dain, *Disordered Minds,* Williamsburg, The Colonial Williamsburg Foundation (distributed by the University Press of Virginia), 1971.

21. M. Friedman, and A. J. Schwartz, *A Monetary History of the United States, 1867–1960,* Princeton, N.J., Princeton University Press, 1963.

22. Proposition 13 called for a 57% reduction in property taxes and was supported by a 2 to 1 vote in California on June 13, 1978. Its impact was mainly on schools, libraries, street sanitation, and community services. See *Time,* June 19, 1978, p. 9.

23. R. R. Grinker, Sr., "Psychiatry rides madl. in all directions," *Archives of General Psychiatry,* vol. 10, March, 1964, p. 228.

3. A glance at history

1. S. T. Rand, *Dictionary of the Language of the Micmac Indians,* Halifax, Nova Scotia Printing Co., 1888.

2. J. Brøndsted, *The Vikings,* Harmondsworth, England, Penguin Books, 1965.

3. F. J. Braceland, *The Institute of Living,* Hartford, Conn., The Institute of Living, 1972.

4. G. Zilboorg and G. W. Henry, *A Historical Medical Psychology,* New York, W. W. Norton, 1941.

5. E. H. Achernecht, *Rudolf Ludwig Karl Virchow, Doctor, Statesman, Anthropologist,* Madison, University of Wisconsin Press, 1953.

6. This picture emerges from the following sources: J. S. Bockhoven, *Moral Treatment in Community Mental Health,* New York, Springer, 1972; R. B. Caplan, *Psychiatry and the Community in Nineteenth-Century America,* New York, Basic Books, 1969; N. Dain, *Disordered Minds,* Williamsburg, The Colonial Williamsburg Foundation (distributed by the University Press of Virginia), 1971; G. N. Grob, *Mental Institutions in America: Social Policy to 1875,* New York, The Free Press, 1973; P. Pinel, *Traité Médico-Philosophique sur l'Alienation Mentale,* Paris, 1809.

7. Grob, *Mental Institutions in America.*

8. Caplan, *Psychiatry and the Community,* p. 100.

9. Pinel, *Traité Médico-Philosophique,* pp. 248, 251.

10. Braceland, *The Institute of Living,* pp. 42–50; Dain, *Disordered Minds,* pp. 44–6, 115–16, 118; Grob, *Mental Institutions in America,* pp. 68–9, 98, 165, 182–5.

11. Dain, *Disordered Minds,* pp. 113–16, 140–60; Grob, *Mental Institutions in America,* pp. 234–43, 263–4, 307–8.

12. According to one biographer, there is reason to believe that Darwin's well-known invalidism was caused by his unhappiness over the implications of his discovery. See Ralph Colp, *To Be an Invalid: The Illness of Charles Darwin,* Chicago, University of Chicago Press, 1977.

13. E. W. Fornell, *The Unhappy Medium,* Austin, The University of Texas Press, 1964, p. 79.

14. M. Friedman and A. J. Schwartz, *A Monetary History of the United States, 1867–1960,* Princeton, N.J., Princeton University Press, 1963; S. A. Saunders, *Studies in the Economy of the Maritime Provinces,* Toronto, The Macmillan Co. of Canada, 1939.

15. Grob, *Mental Institutions in America,* pp. 231–43; E. Jarvis, *Insanity and Idiocy in Massachusetts: Report of the Commission on Lunacy, 1855,* Cambridge, Mass., pp. 57–68 (Reprinted, Cambridge, Mass., Harvard University Press, 1971).

16. Pliny Earle, *The Curability of Insanity: A Series of Studies,* Philadelphia, J. B. Lippincott, 1887, pp. 22–4 (reprinted, New York, Arno Press and *The New York Times,* 1972). For an opposing view, see Jacques M. Quen, "Asylum psychiatry, neurology, social work and mental hygiene: An exploratory study in interprofessional history, *Journal of the History of the Behavioral Sciences,* vol. 13, 1977, pp. 4–5.

17. Bockhoven, *Moral Treatment in Community Mental Health,* p. 55.

18. Grob, *Mental Institutions in America,* pp. 310–19.

19. Grob, *Mental Institutions in America,* p. 69.

20. Dain, *Disordered Minds,* pp. 152–5, 158; Grob, *Mental Institutions in America,* pp. 211–19.

21. The term *sentiment* is employed throughout this book in a technical sense to mean a union of affective and cognitive processes. Words such as *opinion* and *value* cover a part of the same ground. Every sentiment is therefore a feeling about something, but no implication of *sentimental* is intended. For a discussion of the concept and an explication of its usefulness, see Alexander H. Leighton, *My Name is Legion: Foundations for a Theory of Man in Relation to Culture,* New York, Basic Books, 1959, pp. 26–8, 226–75, 395–420.

22. Inasmuch as the story of the soldiers' rum is engaging and has been mentioned by several writers, it seemed worth verifying. The proposal was made in a letter from Charles Laurence, governor of Nova Scotia, to the Lords of Trade on December 5, 1753; it was approved by their lordships in a reply on March 4, 1754. Public Archives of Nova Scotia, PANS, RG1, Vol. 36, Document No. 2 and PANS, RG1, Vol. 29, No. 25, Whitehall Dispatches.

23. M. H. L. Grant, "Historical background of the Nova Scotia Hospital, Dartmouth, and the Victoria General Hospital, Halifax," *The Nova Scotia Medical Bulletin,* vol. 16, May 1937, pp. 255, 257. In considering these matters, it is well to recall that differential diagnosis of mental illnesses was very little developed at this time.

24. Grant, "Historical background of the Nova Scotia Hospital"; H. M. Hurd, F. W. Drewry, R. Dewey, C. W. Pilgrim, G. A. Blumer, and T. J. W. Burgess, *The Institutional Care of the Insane in the United States and Canada,* Baltimore, The Johns Hopkins University Press, Vol. 1, 1916, pp. 481–2, 549–50, Vol. 4, 1917, pp. 101–19 (reprinted, New York, Arno Press, 1973).

Hugh Bell, in a petition to the House of Assembly in 1845, described the problem and the viewpoint he represented in the following words: "That there are now in the Poor's Asylum in the City forty Insane persons, and that according to the general rule which inquiry and observation has established on the subject . . . there are probably two hundred and fifty such cases in the Province. That until very recently such cases have been considered and treated as hopeless, and the unhappy subjects have been viewed as outcasts from Society, and only like inferior animals to be caged and chained and whipped into submission, as if entitled no longer to the characteristics which distinguish from the 'beasts that perish' and as if the link which unites them to the human family were entirely dissolved. The advance of intelligence, of civilization and science have dissipated these gross and misanthropic ideas – have made ashamed of these barbarous practices and have stimulated to efforts in behalf of this class of our suffering fellow beings. In almost every Country in Europe and America, and nearly in every town, Asylums are now provided for their especial benefit and by a system of kindness and sympathy treating them as still of our own species and as intellectual beings, – exciting their love instead of their fear'' (see Grant, "Historical background of the Nova Scotia Hospital," p. 315).

The fact that the mental hospital movement was part of a broader sweep of humanitarian sentiment is illustrated by Dorothea Dix's activities while she was visiting Nova Scotia. With the aid of Hugh Bell, she visited Sable Island and later took part in improving greatly its life-saving resources. Loss of life from shipwreck was a common occurrence at this time, and Sable Island, a crescent of sand about 100 miles from the coast, was notorious as "the graveyard of the Atlantic." Nova Scotia had for some years maintained a beach patrol and life-saving station on this remote spot, and it is possible that Dix was attracted to the island by rumors that mentally ill persons were being sent there as a cheap form of custody. Apparently, she did not find this to be the case but did discover that the life-saving team suffered from inadequate equipment. Chance gave her a good opportunity to make observations about this, as a wreck occurred while she was there and she was a witness to the rescue efforts. It would almost seem that fate recognized her presence with an added touch, for the captain of the wrecked ship turned out to be insane. (See R. Blake, "Dorothea Dix – a forgotten samaritan in Nova Scotia," *The Maritime Advocate and Busy East,* May 1952, pp. 11–16.)

25. E. C. Purdy, *History of the Nova Scotia Hospital,* unpublished manuscript completed in 1976 and based on the hospital's annual reports beginning in 1858.

26. Clyde Marshall, *Report of the Inspector of Humane Institutions: Seventieth Annual Report,* Halifax, printed by order of the Legislature, Queens Printer, 1956, pp. 5–6.

27. Marshall, *Report of the Inspector of Humane Institutions,* p. 7.

28. Marshall, *Report of the Inspector of Humane Institutions,* p. 11.

29. Marshall, *Report of the Inspector of Humane Institutions,* p. 16.

30. Hurd et al., *The Institutional Care of the Insane,* p. 482. This is an appendix that gives, in its entirety, Dix's *Memorial to the Honorable the Legislative Assembly of the Province of Nova Scotia, and its Dependencies.*

31. "Report on public charities for the year ending 30th September, 1900," *Nova Scotia House of Assembly Journals, Appendix No. 3 (A)* Halifax, 1901, p. 2. It might be noted that the 40 percent figure is probably somewhat inflated, as it seems likely that some of the "cured" were from among those admitted prior to the start of the year being reported.

32. "Report on public charities for the year ending 30th September, 1900," *Appendix 3 (B),* pp. 18–50.

33. Grob, *Mental Institutions in America,* pp. 182, 306–8.

34. Questions about the nature and functioning of the mind were of great concern to writers in the romantic period that spanned the end of the eighteenth and the early part of the nineteenth centuries. In consequence, we may suppose that the topic was drawn to the attention of literate and thinking people more generally. One of the issues was whether the mind is a passive receptor that accumulates impressions imposed upon it by the surrounding world or an active projector whereby the process of perception is both receptive and creative. According to the romantic view, as Coleridge put it, man is a creature "of eye, ear, touch, and taste in contact with external nature, and informing the senses from the mind and not compounding a mind out of the senses." The opposed view was the tabula rasa orientation, now associated with the name of Locke, but widely popular in the eighteenth century and harking back to Plato.

Viewing the mind as something which has its own thrust, like a growing plant, was part of a theory to explain the creative process in artists, especially poets, and was approached through comparative analysis of their productions and their life stories. There are many points of similarity between this and a clinician's approach to understanding the delusions, hallucinations, and emotions of a patient in terms of personality, environment, and life story. Literary philosophers and the poets themselves tried to explain how the productions of a poet arose from the mind interacting with experiences. It appears that they conceptualized, before clinicians did, the importance of repression in such matters. In Keble's words (written for his lectures at Oxford between 1832 and 1841), "Poetry is the indirect expression . . . of some overpowering emotion . . . the direct indulgence whereof is somehow repressed." Drawing attention to the ancient notion that poetic inspiration is a form of insanity, Keble suggests that it is, rather, "a safety valve preserving men from actual madness." Still earlier, there were also adumbrations of the unconscious by Schelling and Richter. Richter speaks of it as the source of dreams and says the poetic genius is "in more than one sense a sleepwalker." (See M. H. Abrams, *The Mirror and the Lamp: Romantic Theory and the Critical Condition*, New York, Oxford University Press, 1953, pp. 58, 145, 147, 211–212.)

There were, however, other more direct and personal events that forced questions about the mind and how it functions on the attention of these poets, philosophers, and critics. William Cowper (1731–1800) had recurrent attacks of what was apparently psychotic depression throughout his life, in one of which he made a serious suicidal attempt. During the first of these episodes, he spent eighteen months in an asylum and during the others lived under sheltered conditions. John Clare, the "Northamptonshire Peasant Poet" (1793–1864), was even more severely impaired than Cowper by some kind of psychotic illness and spent the last thirty years of his life in an asylum.

The question of whether the visions of William Blake (1757–1827) were pathological is a matter of debate that may never be settled. Nevertheless, the fact that the issue was discussed during Blake's lifetime indicates contemporary puzzling over creativity and madness. According to the Encyclopedia Britannica, Robert Southey regarded him as insane, although those closer to him thought otherwise.

Charles Lamb (1775–1834), who personally knew Coleridge, Hazlitt, Wordsworth, and other leading writers of his day, had a life dominated by mental illness. In 1796, his sister Mary murdered their mother and was judged insane. Lamb devoted the rest of his life to her care, doing his best to keep her out of asylums as much as possible. He, himself, also had an episode of some kind during which he spent a short time in an asylum.

Samuel Taylor Coleridge (1772–1834) had a dependency on opium which troubled him and led eventually to his retiring into the home of James Gillman in Highgate, where he spent almost all of the last eighteen years of his life, socially isolated though still writing.

The turbulent politics in England during this same period were further perturbed by recurrent episodes of mental illness in a politically active and strong-willed king, George III. The first disturbance was in 1765, and the last and permanent one began in 1811. Though the insanity of the king is well known, less remembered is the fact that Lord Chatham, while head of the government, was incapacitated by a severe depression for almost two years, 1767–1769 (Manfred S. Guttmacher, *America's Last King: An Interpretation of the Madness of George III*, New York, Charles Scribner's Sons, 1941, pp. 93–99). This occurrence at the beginning of George's reign is matched by another, even greater, disturbance to the government shortly after his death. On August 12, 1822, Castlereagh, Britain's great political architect of Europe's coalition against Napoleon and subsequently the leader of conservative policies at home, committed suicide with a penknife in what his doctors and his friend the Duke of Wellington said was an episode of mental illness.

There is reason to believe, therefore, that politics as well as literature gave many people highly specific causes to ponder on the nature of the mind and the forces that can lead either to its being productive and great or to its becoming unhinged.

35. A short account of the relationship between neurologists and asylum superintendents is given by Quen and a longer treatment is provided by Sickerman. Quen, "Asylum Psychiatry, Neurology, Social Work and Mental Hygiene," pp. 3–11; Barbara Sickerman, *The Quest for Mental Health in America 1880–1917,* doctoral thesis, Columbia University, New York, 1967, reproduced and distributed by University Microfilms International, Ann Arbor, Mich., 1979, particularly pp. 35–8, 56–64, 176–7.

36. W. A. Hammond, "The non-asylum treatment of the insane," *Transactions of the Medical Society of the State of New York,* Syracuse, 1879, p. 281.

37. S. W. Mitchell, "Address before the fiftieth annual meeting of the American Medico-Psychological Association," *Journal of Nervous and Mental Diseases,* vol. 21, 1894, p. 426.

38. Most of this discussion of Meyer is based on recollections from four years as a resident at the Henry Phipps Psychiatric Clinic when Meyer was professor of psychiatry and chief of the service. For a description of psychobiology and Meyer's terminology for dealing with mental illnesses, see Adolf Meyer, "Leading Concepts of Psychobiology (Ergasiology) and of Psychiatry (Ergasiatry)," in Eunice E. Winters, ed., *The Collected Papers of Adolf Meyer,* Vol. 3, Baltimore, The Johns Hopkins University Press, 1952, pp. 285–314.

39. Abrams, *The Mirror and the Lamp,* p. 175.

40. In this book, *scientific practice* refers to care-giving procedures that utilize already available scientific knowledge but that are not, in themselves, concerned with scientific discovery or testing. *Scientific research* refers to the discovery and testing of new knowledge by means of scientific procedures. The two generally differ considerably in the technical skills and modes of thinking required and are, therefore, often conducted by different individuals. For this reason, they should not be lumped together. See J. C. Cassel and A. H. Leighton, "Epidemiology and Mental Health," in Stephen E. Goldstein, ed., *Mental Health Considerations in Public Health* (Chapter 4), Washington, D.C., National Institute of Mental Health, U.S. Department of Health, Education, and Welfare, 1969.

41. For examples, see Adolf Meyer, "The Meaning of Maturity," and "Where Should We Attack the Problem of Mental Defect and Mental Disease?" in Winters, ed., *The Collected Papers of Adolf Meyer,* Vol. 4, pp. 190–7, 425–34.

42. Chester R. Burns, "Diseases versus Healths: Some Legacies in the Philosophies of Modern Medical Science," in H. Tristram Englehardt, Jr., and Stuart F. Spicker, eds., *Evaluation and Explanation in the Biomedical Sciences,* Boston, D. Reidel, 1974, pp. 35, 40.

43. Sickerman, *The Quest for Mental Health in America,* p. 286.

44. Clifford Whittingham Beers, *A Mind that Found Itself: An Autobiography,* Garden City, N.Y., Doubleday, 1970 (reprinted).

45. Adolf Meyer, "Organization of Community Facilities for Prevention, Care and Treatment of Nervous and Mental Disease," in Winters, ed., *The Collected Papers of Adolf Meyer,* Vol. 4, p. 266.

46. William A. White, "Underlying concepts in mental hygiene," *Mental Hygiene,* vol. 1, no. 1, 1917, p. 14.

47. White, "Underlying concepts in mental hygiene," p. 15.

48. Quoted by Barbara A. Dreyer, "Adolf Meyer and mental hygiene: An ideal for public health," *American Journal of Public Health,* vol. 66, no. 10, 1976, pp. 998–1003.

49. According to Sickerman (*The Quest for Mental Health in America,* p. 291) these were, in addition to Beers and Meyer, William James, Julia Lathrop; Lewellyn F. Barker and Frederick Peterson (two neurologists of distinction); August Hoch; Rev. Anson Phelps Stokes, Jr. (Secretary of Yale University); Russell Chittenden (a lay physiologist at the Sheffield Scientific School of Yale); Jacob Gould Schurman (president of Cornell University); Marcus Marks (a merchant); and Horace Fletcher (a popular writer on nutrition and health). Other early members of the national committee were Dr. William Welch, Jane Addams, Cardinal Gibbons (the leading Catholic prelate in America), Irving Fisher, and Charles W. Eliot (president of Harvard).

50. Sickerman, *The Quest for Mental Health in America,* pp. 306, 310, 312.

51. Sickerman, *The Quest for Mental Health in America,* pp. 314. Beers's view of the scope of mental hygiene was not confined to individuals prone to be carried away by enthusiasm. It was supported by some of psychiatry's most distinguished professionals and major contributors. This can be illustrated by quoting C. Macfie Campbell, professor of psychiatry at Harvard, chairman of the Committee on Education of the National Committee for Mental Hygiene, and former trainee of Adolf Meyer: "A disorder is a mental disorder if its roots are mental. A headache indicates a mental disorder if it comes because one is dodging something disagreeable. A pain in the back is a mental disorder if its persistence is due to discouragement and a feeling of uncertainty and a desire to have sick benefit, rather than to put one's back into one's work. Sleeplessness is a mental disorder if its basis lies in personal worries and emotional tangles. Many mental reactions are indications of poor mental health, although they are not usually classified as mental disorders. Discontent with one's environment may be a mental disorder, if its cause lie, not in some external situation, but in personal failure to deal with one's emotional problems. Suspicion, distrust, misinterpretation, are mental disorders when they are the disguised expression of repressed longings, into which the patient has no clear insight. Stealing sometimes indicates a mental disorder, the odd expression of underlying conflicts in the patient's nature. The feeling of fatigue sometimes represents, not overwork, but discouragement, inability to meet situations, lack of interest in the opportunities available. Unsociability, marital incompatibility, alcoholism, an aggressive and embittered social attitude, may all indicate a disorder of the mental balance, which may be open to modification. Acute phenomena characterized by unreasoning emotional reactions, such as lynching and other mob reactions, waves of popular suspicion sweeping over a country, may be looked upon as transitory disorders. The same factors that are involved in these familiar reactions play an important part in the development of insanity" (from Beers, *A Mind that Found Itself,* rev. 5th ed., 1921, pp. 301–2, taken by him from an article by Campbell in *Mental Hygiene,* July 1921).

52. J. C. Perry, "Four Twentieth-Century Themes in Community Mental Health Programs," in Burton H. Kaplan, Robert N. Wilson, and Alexander H. Leighton, eds., *Further Explorations in Social Psychiatry,* New York, Basic Books, 1976, p. 50.

53. See N. Ridenour, "A Nucleus but No Boundary," Chapter XIII in *Mental Health in the United States,* Cambridge, Mass., Harvard University Press (for the Commonwealth Fund), 1961.

54. This summary is based on the following sources: G. E. Hart, "Early private relief in Nova Scotia," *Welfare News,* vol. 2, no. 2., July 1951, pp. 4–5; G. E. Hart, "The Halifax Poor Man's Friend Society, 1820–27, an early experiment," *The Canadian Historical Review,* vol. 34, no. 2, June 1953, pp. 109–22; T. H. Raddall, *Halifax, Warden of the North,* Toronto, McClelland and Stewart, 1948, Chapters 18–23; Department of Welfare, "Welfare Services in Nova Scotia," Public Archives of Nova Scotia, HV76, N93, W44, 1965, pp. 19–39.

In the early part of the nineteenth century, Halifax was a city of contrast between the haves and have-nots, especially during the years of depression that followed the end of the Napoleonic wars and the War of 1812. Moreover, many of the have-nots lived up the hill above the opulent area with "its fine mansions and shady willows." As a result, "all the seepage of that wallowing slum . . . came down with the rains into the ornate gardens and spotless kitchens . . . The town was not so much a whited sepulchre as a gilded chamberpot" (Raddall, *Halifax, Warden of the North,* p. 159).

According to Hart ("Early Private Relief"), the Poor Man's Friend Society was preceded by a Society for the Relief of the Poor. He says that during the winter of 1809 "the cold was so intense and the snow so deep that outdoor employment came to a standstill. By February many families were about to perish from lack of food and fuel. Fire and disease were fearsome giants which laid their frequent victims prostrate and impoverished their survivors." As a result, a number of "business and professional men of Halifax met early in February to consider 'the most effectual means for relieving the wants of the Poor at this inclement season' and they resolved that those present should immediately form themselves into a Society for the Relief of the Poor. Each member was to subscribe half a dollar a week during the 'six winter months' and a quarter-dollar a week during the rest of the year. There were fifty-three members at first including the Bishop of Nova Scotia, judges, doctors, clergymen, merchants, and others. A treasurer was named and a committee of two clergymen, two merchants, a physician, and a member of the legislature was set up 'to investigate the cases of all persons applying for relief, and to afford them such assistance as their necessities might appear to require.' The committee spent one-half of the £640 at its disposal in providing cordwood to the 'industrious poor.' It gave out almost £100 worth of food – sugar, tea, rice, flour, and bread. It used some of the money for blankets, shoes, stockings, baizes, and linen, paid some out for rents, and appropriated a few pounds for nursing, wines and medicines in a smallpox case. It helped sundry poor Indians and supplied board for a man from Chezzetcook with a cancered lip. It provided work instead of relief when it could, for it paid forty pounds to twenty-eight poor labourers for clearing the gutters and drains of ice and snow in the winter of 1809. Nor were its charitable activities confined to the town of Halifax. £120 was distributed 'to 84 persons in great distress with sick families, others burnt out, etc., in the towns of Halifax, Dartmouth, Preston, Chezzetcook (sic), St. Mary's Sisiboo, Shelburne, Digby, Lawrencetown, Windsor Road, etc.' "

In March 1811, the society for some reason considered its work done and proceeded to pass quietly out of existence. This was, to say the least, optimistic. Again, according to Hart ("The Halifax Poor Man's Friend Society," pp. 110–12, 119, 123), the poor of Halifax were "caught in the vise of hard times created by the Napoleonic Wars; hard times tightened by colonial trade restrictions, by farming tied to supplying the armed forces, and by lack of industry; hard times made crushing by early frost, too much rain, and a plague of field mice. So widespread was the destitution resulting from crop failures that in the years immediately after the Wars the government spent more than ten thousand pounds on farm relief. Halifax saw all kinds of misery. A thousand poor Scotch and Irish immigrants arrived in 1816 and more than two thousand in each of the following three years. Large bands of Irishmen came from Newfoundland. Men tramped in from the rest of the province looking for work. The town of ten thousand people could provide them with neither employment nor decent housing."

The Society for the Relief of the Poor was followed in 1817 by an Association for the Relief of the Labouring Poor, and this, in turn, by the Poor Man's Friend Society. Its leader was Walter Bromley, "a retired army paymaster who had served under the Duke of Wellington and the founder and master of the Royal Acadian School for the poor children of Halifax." The group of citizens who met at the Royal Acadian School on February 17, 1820, agreed on a constitution for the new Society. The members were to pay an initial fee of twenty shillings, give a shilling a month, and act as visitors of the poor. They reserved the right to choose yearly from among themselves a managing committee of twenty men. A subcommittee of four members was to meet once a week to consider the cases reported by the visitors and to conduct any business delegated to it by the managing committee. Each visitor was obliged to inquire into needy cases in his ward; if necessary, he was to grant aid of not more than five shillings until the subcommittee could review the facts. He was required to collect the monthly subscription from the members in his ward. He must encourage journeymen and servants to give sixpence a month, telling them that through sickness or other adversity they might some day need help from the Society. After the meeting the Society circulated two thousand copies of an address to the public, urging citizens not to give alms to young beggars and describing its plan to assist, after careful investigation, 'every case of suffering humanity within the precincts of the town.' It stated that aid would be given in kind because experience had shown that cash relief encouraged vice. Its liberal rule of eligibility was printed in italics: '. . . no distinction will be made on account of the nation, sect, or party, to which the sufferer may belong; real distress, wherever found, will be the only recommendation required.' The new committee divided the town into seventeen wards and appointed two visitors to each. The Society reported at its first annual meeting in December 1820, that it had helped 4,213 men, women, and children; it had provided wood, clothing, bedding, and food, amounting in all to £400. The visitors had enforced the rule that parents would not receive help if their children begged. The report expressed regret that the Society was short of money because wage-earners had not contributed a small part of their income as often as had been expected and some subscribers had not paid."

At the end of seven years, the Poor Man's Friend Society also faded, even though there were soon new waves of impoverished immigrants and swarms of beggars. The rise and fade pattern is a notable feature of all the humanitarian associations I have reviewed as background for this study. The reasons for the fading were doubtless multiple, but it is evident that among them were economic fluctuations, decrease in funding, loss of members, departure of leaders (e.g., Bromley went back to England), and ideological opposition that became intense and bitter. Although stoutly defended by some, the society was denounced by others for encouraging poverty by helping the poor and thus preventing "the natural checks to population to act free and without control." In his conclusion, ("The Halifax Poor Man's Friend Society,") Hart says, "While the people of that generation emphasized the personal causes of poverty, the Society, to its lasting credit, recognized and proclaimed some of the social factors in destitution. It reminded the public more than once that reverses of fortune might come to any one and that many persons were reduced to a state of hunger and starvation by illness and a general condition of unemployment. Its committee of industry reported that the unemployed men whom it had interviewed were "perfectly willing to work." It vigorously attempted to initiate a savings bank and a programme of employment because it realized the importance of self-help as a partial solution of the plight of the poor. Unfortunately the doctrine of laissez-faire and the moralizing objection to poor relief as voiced by the Malthusians destroyed the Society just when it was evolving procedures for the humane and enlightened treatment of the poor – in contrast with the current handling of them as near-criminals."

As one final note of incidental interest, an active member of the Poor Man's Friend Society when it was formed in 1820 was the same Hugh Bell who later played such a leading part in founding the Nova Scotia Hospital. Another was Samuel Cunard, founder of the Cunard Steamship Line.

55. This summary is based on the following sources: Minutes of the Halifax local of the Council of Women, 1894–1947, Public Archives of Nova Scotia MG, 20, vol. 535, nos. 1–13, 1894–1947; Scrapbook of the Halifax local of the Council of Women, 1908–1917, Public Archives of Nova Scotia MG, 20, vol. 535, no. 10; Minute Book of the Nova Scotia League for Protection of the Feeble Minded and the Nova Scotia Society for Mental Hygiene, 1908–38, courtesy of Mental Health – Nova Scotia [The Nova Scotia Mental Health Association], Halifax, Nova Scotia; The Nova Scotia Society for Mental Hygiene, 1948 (pamphlet issued at time of the fortieth anniversary, outlining the organization's history, on file in the office of Mental Health – Nova Scotia [the Nova Scotia Mental Health Association], Halifax: "An Act to incorporate the Nova Scotia Society for Mental Hygiene," The Statutes of Nova Scotia, Halifax, King's Printer, 1931.

It is apparent from the above minutes that these later organizations also experienced marked fluctuations in activities and interest on the part of members. For example, the minute book of the Council of Women shows nothing for the years 1899–1902, 1910–11, and 1930–1. The League for the Protection of the Feeble Minded had no meetings from 1914 to 1919 and from 1922 to 1923.

56. This summary is based on the following sources: Minute Book of the Nova Scotia League for the Protection of the Feeble Minded and the Nova Scotia Society for Mental Hygiene, 1908–38; *The Nova Scotia Society for Mental Hygiene* pamphlet; "Samuel H. Prince," in B. M. Greene, ed., *Who's Who in Canada,* Toronto, International Press, 1956–7; *Report of the Royal Commission Concerning Mentally Deficient Persons in Nova Scotia, 1927,* Halifax, King's Printer, 1927.

57. R. O. Jones, professor of psychiatry emeritus, Faculty of Medicine, Dalhousie University, personal communication, 1976.

58. Jones, personal communication, 1976.

59. H. A. Cotton, "The etiology and treatment of the so-called functional psychoses, summary of results based upon the experience of four years," *American Journal of Psychiatry,* vol. 79, October 1922, pp. 157–94; H. A. Bunker, "American Psychiatric Literature during the Past One Hundred Years," in *One Hundred Years of American Psychiatry,* published for the American Psychiatric Association, New York, Columbia University Press, 1944, p. 247; W. Malamud, "The History of Psychiatric Therapies," in *One Hundred Years of American Psychiatry,* pp. 308–9, 311.

60. Again, most of this discussion is based on recollections from four years as a resident under Meyer. For elaboration, see Meyer, "Leading Concepts of Psychobiology."

61. J. C. Smuts, *Holism and Evolution,* London, Macmillan, 1927.

62. Alexander H. Leighton, "Introduction," in Eunice E. Winters, ed., *The Collected Papers of Adolf Meyer,* Vol. 4, Baltimore, The Johns Hopkins University Press, 1952, p. xxii.

63. P. A. Robinson, *The Freudian Left,* New York, Harper & Row, 1969.

64. A. I. Hallowell, *Culture and Experience,* Philadelphia, University of Pennsylvania Press, 1955, p. 434.

65. A. H. Leighton and J. M. Hughes (Murphy), "Cultures as Causative of Mental Disorder," in *Causes of Mental Disorders: A Review of Epidemiological Knowledge,* New York, Milbank Memorial Fund, 1961, pp. 341–65.

66. A. Kardiner, *The Individual and His Society,* New York, Columbia University Press, 1939.

67. M. K. Opler, *Culture, Psychiatry, and Human Values,* Springfield, Ill., Charles C. Thomas, 1956.

68. G. H. Mead, *Mind, Self and Society,* Chicago, University of Chicago Press, 1934.

69. R. E. L. Faris and H. W. Dunham, *Mental Disorder in Urban Areas,* Chicago, University of Chicago Press, 1939.

70. W. L. Warner and P. S. Lunt, *The Social Life of a Modern Community,* New Haven, Yale University Press, 1941.

71. R. R. Grinker, and J. P. Spiegel, *Men under Stress,* New York, Blakiston (McGraw-Hill), 1945.

72. D. C. Lewis, and B. Engle, eds., *Wartime Psychiatry,* New York, Oxford University Press, 1954.

73. W. Sargant, and E. Slater, "Acute war neuroses," *The Lancet,* vol. 2, 1940, pp. 1–2.

74. Lewis and Engle, *Wartime Psychiatry,* Chapters 6, 9, 13. For a discussion of environmental conditions that reduce rates of psychological casualties in battle, see pp. 563–4, 873–4.

75. See, for example, A. H. Leighton, *The Governing of Men,* Princeton, N.J., Princeton University Press, 1945; A. H. Leighton, *Human Relations in a Changing World,* New

York, E. P. Dutton, 1949; Office of Strategic Services (H. A. Murray), *Assessment of Men: Selection of Personnel for the Office of Strategic Services,* New York, Rinehart, 1948; S. A. Stouffer, A. A. Lumsdaine, M. H. Lumsdaine, R. M. Williams, Jr., M. B. Smith, I. L. Janis, S. A. Star, and L. S. Cottrell, Jr., *The American Soldier, Combat and Its Aftermath,* vol. 2, Princeton, N.J., Princeton University Press, 1949.

76. This summary is based partly on personal recollection and partly on the following sources: Bertram, S. Brown, "The federal mental health program: Past, present, and future," *Hospital and Community Psychiatry,* vol. 27, no. 7, July 1976, p. 512; Henry A. Foley, *Community Mental Health Legislation,* Lexington, Mass., D. C. Heath, 1975, pp. 3–6; Luther E. Woodward, "The Mental Hygiene Movement – More Recent Developments," in Beers, *A Mind that Found Itself, An Autobiography,* rev. ed., pp. 361–2.

77. Elizabeth I. Adamson, "The aim and accomplishments of a health center mental hygiene program," *American Journal of Public Health,* vol. 23, 1933, p. 215.

78. George H. Preston, "The new public psychiatry," *Mental Hygiene,* vol. 31, no. 2, 1947, p. 177.

79. Personal communication from R. C. Hunter to Ralph Kuna, March 1978. Mr. Hunter was one of the participants in the creation of the National Mental Health Foundation. Another participant has told us: "The amalgamation of the Federation and the Committee required a name that carried on the tradition of neither – it was an item in reaching the merger. It was not so much a new identity as a political maneuver that would allow merger."

80. B. Chisholm, "On the march for mental health," *Survey Graphic,* vol. 36, no. 10, October 1947, p. 509.

81. Nova Scotia Commission on Provincial Development and Rehabilitation, Section 4, *Report on Public Welfare Services,* Halifax, King's Printer, 1944, p. 133.

82. In 1947, the title was chief of neuropsychiatry. With time and reorganization, it eventually became administrator of the Psychiatric Mental Health Administration. This transition illustrates some of the trends discussed in the text. *Psychiatric Mental Health* can be interpreted as an effort to adjust to popular trends while at the same time retaining some specificity of meaning. In this book, the label *Mental Health Administration* will be used in order to avoid the confusion that might occur if the titles of different time periods were employed and also to avoid the seeming contradiction and awkwardness of the simultaneous use of *psychiatric* and *mental health.*

83. C. Marshall, "Report of the Chief of the Neuropsychiatric Division," *Annual Report 1946–1947,* Nova Scotia Department of Public Health, Halifax, King's Printer, 1948, pp. 193–4.

84. J. J. Schwab and M. E. Schwab, *Sociocultural Roots of Mental Illness: An Epidemiologic Survey,* New York, Plenum, 1978, pp. 6–7.

85. Lawrence K. Frank, "The Promotion of Mental Health," *Annals of The American Academy of Political and Social Sciences,* vol. 286, no. 36, 1953, p. 170.

4. The formation of a mental health center at mid-century

1. A. Meyer, "Where should we attack the problem of prevention of mental defect and mental disease?", in E. E. Winters, ed., vol. 4, *The Collected Papers of Adolf Meyer,* Baltimore, The Johns Hopkins University Press, 1952, p. 196.

2. In the beginning, the service was called a psychiatric clinic, but as the mental health movement grew, it was renamed as a mental health center. For the sake of simplicity, the latter designation will be used in these pages.

3. Arie Querido, "The shaping of community mental health care," *British Journal of Psychiatry,* vol. 114, 1968, pp. 293–302.

4. E. J. Cleveland and W. D. Longaker, "Neurotic Patterns in the Family," in Alexander H. Leighton, John A. Clausen, and Robert N. Wilson, eds., *Explorations in Social Psychiatry*, New York, Basic Books, 1957, pp. 167–200.

5. Another glance at history

1. W. S. Maclay, "Experiments in mental hospital organization," *The Canadian Medical Association Journal*, vol. 78, no. 12, 1958, pp. 909–16.

2. Joint Commission on Mental Illness and Health, *Action for Mental Health*, New York, Basic Books, 1961, pp. 263–4.

3. Canadian Mental Health Association, *More for the Mind*, Toronto, 1963, p. 40.

4. John F. Kennedy, "Message from the President of the United States relative to mental illness and mental retardation," House of Representatives Document No. 58, 88th Congress, 1st Session, February 5, 1963, p. 3.

5. Henry A. Foley, *Community Mental Health Legislation; The Formative Process*, Lexington, Mass., D. C. Heath, 1975, pp. 126–7.

6. Foley, *Community Mental Health Legislation*, pp. 130, 132.

7. D. F. Musto, "Whatever happened to community mental health?", *Public Interest*, vol. 39, 1975, pp. 53–79.

8. A. A. Stone, "Psychiatry: Dead or alive?", *Harvard Magazine*, December 1976, p. 19. See also R. M. Murray, "A reappraisal of American psychiatry," *The Lancet*, vol. 1, no. 8110, February 3, 1979, pp. 255–8.

9. R. Laing and A. Esterson, *Sanity, Madness, and the Family*, New York, Basic Books, 1964; T. S. Szasz, *The Myth of Mental Illness: Foundation of a Theory of Personal Conduct*, New York, Hoeber-Harper, 1961.

10. E. Goffman, *Asylums: Essays on the Social Situation of Mental Patients and Other Inmates*, Chicago, Aldine, 1962; D. Mechanic, "Some factors in identifying and defining mental illness," *Mental Hygiene*, vol. 46, 1962, p. 68; T. Sarbin, "The Scientific Status of the Mental Illness Metaphor," in S. Plog and R. Edgerton, eds., *Changing Perspectives in Mental Illness*, New York, Holt, Rinehart & Winston, 1969; and T. Scheff, *Being Mentally Ill: A Sociological Theory*, Chicago, Aldine, 1966.

11. Nova Scotia Council of Health, *Health Care in Nova Scotia: A New Direction for the Seventies*, Government of Nova Scotia, 1972, p. 81.

12. Jonathan F. Borus, "Issues critical to the survival of community mental health," *American Journal of Psychiatry*, vol. 135, no. 9, September 1978, pp. 1029–35.

13. Marmur further observes, "It is interesting that some therapists are beginning to herald the birth of a fourth revolution, 'transpersonal psychology,' which encompasses such elements as mysticism, extrasensory perception, precognition, life-after-death, and reincarnation. I shall not discuss this fourth movement except to mention that in some ways it represents a logical extension of the third revolution." Judd Marmur, "Recent trends in psycho-therapy," *American Journal of Psychiatry*, vol. 137, no. 4, April 1980, p. 410. We appear to be on our way back to the spiritualism of the nineteenth century described in Chapter 3.

14. For example, see R. B. Blishen, *Doctors and Doctrines: The Ideology of Medical Care in Canada*, Toronto, University of Toronto Press, 1969; C. B. Chapman and J. M. Talmadge, "Historical and political background of federal health care legislation," *Law and Contemporary Problems*, vol. 35, Spring 1970, pp. 334–47.

15. Blishen, *Doctors and Doctrines*, p. 151.

16. Blishen, *Doctors and Doctrines*, p. 176.

17. David Woods, "Whither general practice?", *Canadian Medical Association Journal*, Vol. 121, September 8, 1979, p. 621.

18. W. McDermott, "General medical care, identification and analysis of alternative approaches," *Hopkins Medical Journal,* vol. 135, November 1974, p. 298.

19. Theodore Roszak, *"The Making of a Counter Culture,"* New York, Doubleday, 1969.

20. J. Kerouac, *On the Road,* New York, Viking Press, 1959; V. Bugliosi, *Helter Skelter,* New York, Bantam Books, 1975.

21. I. Hamilton, *The Children's Crusade,* Toronto, Peter Martin Associates, 1970, p. 8.

22. Hamilton, *The Children's Crusade,* p. 9.

23. Hamilton, *The Children's Crusade,* pp. 22–3.

24. Hamilton, *The Children's Crusade,* p. iv.

25. H. Osmond, "The crisis within," *Psychiatric Annals,* vol. 3, no. 11, November 1972, pp. 59–60.

26. Stone, "Psychiatry: Dead or Alive?", p. 17.

27. Stone, "Psychiatry: Dead or Alive?", pp. 18, 19, 21.

28. J. Herbers, "Unrest in junior high schools," in N. Sheffe, ed., *Student Unrest,* Toronto, McGraw-Hill, 1969, p. 51.

29. A. R. Blackmer, *An Inquiry into Student Unrest in Independent Secondary Schools,* Boston, National Association of Independent Schools, 1970, p. 21.

30. C. Hobart, "The implications of student power for high schools," *Education Canada,* vol. 9, 1969, p. 29.

31. Blackmer, *An Inquiry into Student Unrest,* pp. 23, 25.

32. S. M. Lipset, *Rebellion in the University: A History of Student Activism in America,* London, Routledge & Kegan Paul, 1972, p. 242.

33. Hobart, "The implications of student power for high schools," p. 27; Blackmer, *An Inquiry into Student Unrest,* p. 50.

34. E. Z. Friedenberg, "The high school as a focus of 'student unrest,'" *American Academy of Political and Social Science Annals,* vol. 395, 1971, pp. 117–26.

35. Hobart, "The implications of student power for high schools," p. 29.

36. C. C. Hughes, M. A. Tremblay, R. N. Rapport, and A. H. Leighton, *People of Cove and Woodlot,* New York, Basic Books, 1960, pp. 386, 433.

37. P. Boyer and S. Nissenbaum, *Salem Possessed: The Social Origins of Witchcraft,* Cambridge, Mass., Harvard University Press, 1974. For a picture of tensions in Sudbury, Massachusetts and other New England towns, see S. C. Powell, *Puritan Village: The Formation of a New England Town,* Middletown, Conn., Connecticut Wesleyan University Press, 1963, pp. 107–10, 116–38.

38. W. Kornhauser, "Power and Participation in the Local Community," *Health Education Monographs,* No. 6, 1959. Reprinted in R. L. Warner, ed., *Perspectives on the American Community: A Book of Readings,* Chicago, Rand McNally, 1966, p. 489.

39. Kornhauser, "Power and Participation in the Local Community," pp. 490, 491, 494.

40. J. S. Coleman, "The Dynamics of Community Controversy," in *Community Conflict,* New York, The Free Press, 1957. Reprinted in Warner, *Perspectives on the American Community,* p. 543.

41. Coleman, "The Dynamics of Community Controversy," p. 550.

6. The Bristol Centre: staff

1. Canadian Mental Health Association, *More for the Mind,* Toronto, Canadian Mental Health Association, 1963.

2. For a summary of the methods used and a breakdown in terms of diagnostic types, see J. M. Murphy, "Continuities in community based psychiatric epidemiology," *Archives of General Psychiatry,* vol. 37, 1980, pp. 1215–23.

3. The Centre was asked by the chairperson of the hospital board to write a proposal and job description for a hospital social worker, but it did not respond.

4. U.S. Department of Health, Education and Welfare, *Concepts of Community Psychiatry,* Washington, D.C., U.S. Government Printing Office, 1965.

5. S. M. Lipset, *Rebellion in the University: A History of Student Activism in America,* London, Routledge & Kegan Paul, 1972. The phrase in our text is one quoted by Lipset from Richard Blum (p. 111).

6. A. H. Leighton and A. Longaker, "The Psychiatric Clinic as a Community Innovation," in A. H. Leighton, J. A. Clausen, and R. N. Wilson, eds., *Explorations in Social Psychiatry,* New York, Basic Books, 1957, pp. 366–82.

7. E. J. Cleveland and W. D. Longaker, "Neurotic Patterns in the Family," in Leighton, Clausen, and Wilson, eds., *Explorations in Social Psychiatry.*

8. Cleveland and Longaker, "Neurotic Patterns in the Family," p. 178.

9. The reader will recall that the Stirling County Study moved from Cornell to Harvard in 1966.

10. Quoted by R. G. Blishen, *Doctors and Doctrines: The Ideology of Medical Care in Canada,* Toronto, University of Toronto Press, 1969, p. 130.

11. Blishen, *Doctors and Doctrines,* p. 57.

12. *Annual Report of the Nova Scotia Department of Public Health,* 1959, p. 115.

13. Blishen, *Doctors and Doctrines,* pp. 88, 139.

14. Adolf Meyer, "Spontaneity," in Eunice E. Winters, ed., *The Collected Papers of Adolf Meyer,* vol. 4, Baltimore, The Johns Hopkins University Press, 1952, pp. 460–83.

15. A. R. Blackmer, *An Inquiry into Student Unrest in Independent Secondary Schools,* Boston, National Association of Independent Schools, 1970, p. 11.

7. The Bristol Centre: Board of Directors

1. The substance of this charge was expressed many times in discussions held before and during the formation of the Board. It was never written down as a single coherent statement but appeared in parts of three documents: the Board's *Memorandum of Association;* the Board's *Bylaws;* and the Mental Health Administration's *Policies and Regulations with Regard to Grants-in-Aid to Community Mental Health Boards.* (Extracts of these documents are reproduced in Appendix A.)

2. A more extended account of these points may be found in A. H. Leighton and A. Longaker, "The Psychiatric Clinic as a Community Innovation," in A. H. Leighton, J. A. Clausen, and R. N. Wilson, eds., *Explorations in Social Psychiatry,* New York, Basic Books, 1957, pp. 365–85.

3. Richard Blum, quoted in S. M. Lipset, *Rebellion in the University: A History of Student Activism in America,* London, Routledge & Kegan Paul, 1972, p. 111.

4. A. Longaker and W. D. Longaker, "The Social Relationships of a Community Mental Health Centre" (review of the first five years of the Bristol Centre). An unpublished report prepared for the Stirling County Study, 1959, with support from the Russell Sage Foundation.

5. "Report of the Scientific Planning Committee of the Nova Scotia Society for Mental Hygiene," November 1954. Made available through the courtesy of Mental Health Nova Scotia (Nova Scotia Mental Health Association).

6. A. C. K. Hallock and W. T. Vaughan "Community organization: A dynamic component of community mental health practice," *American Journal of Orthopsychiatry,* vol. 26, no. 4, 1956, pp. 691–708.

7. R. Bunker and J. Adair, *The First Look at Strangers,* New Brunswick, N.J., Rutgers University Press, 1959; C. C. Hughes, *An Eskimo Village in the Modern World,* Ithaca, N.Y., Cornell University Press, 1960; A. H. Leighton, *Governing of Men,* Princeton, N.J., Princeton University Press, 1945; A. H. Leighton and D. C. Leighton, *The Navaho Door,*

Cambridge, Mass., Harvard University Press, 1944; A. H. Leighton, *Human Relations in a Changing World*, New York, E. P. Dutton, 1949; T. T. Sasaki, *Fruitland, New Mexico, a Navaho Community in Transition*, Ithaca, N.Y. Cornell University Press, 1960; E. H. Spicer, ed., *Human Problems in Technological Change: A Casebook*, New York, Russell Sage Foundation, 1952.

8. A. R. Holmberg, "The Research and Development Approach to Change: Participant Intervention in the Field," in R. N. Adams, ed., *Human Organization Research: Field Relations and Techniques*, Homewood, Ill., The Dorsey Press, 1960; M. E. Opler, "The Creek Town and the Problem of Creek Indian Political Reorganization," in E. H. Spicer, ed., *Human Problems in Technological Change: A Casebook*, New York, Russell Sage Foundation, 1952, pp. 165–80; W. F. Whyte, "The social role of the settlement house," *Applied Anthropology*, vol. 1, no. 1, 1941, pp. 14–19. These articles constitute examples from the works of these authors. Their ideas were mainly transmitted to the Stirling County Study through personal contact, consultations, and conferences, and were exceedingly influential.

9. See Charles Loomis and D. Ensminger, "Governmental administration and informal local groups," *Applied Anthropology*, vol. 1, no. 2, 1942, pp. 41–62; and I. T. Sanders, "The folk approach in extension work," *Applied Anthropology*, vol. 2, no. 4, 1943, pp. 1–10.

10. C. C. Hughes, M. A. Tremblay, R. N. Rapport, and A. H. Leighton, *People of Cove and Woodlot*, New York, Basic Books, 1960.

11. E. J. Cleveland, personal communication, 1977.

12. Stated by the head of the Mental Health Administration in a meeting with Centre staff on May 2, 1951; see also "Report of the Scientific Planning Committee of the Nova Scotia Society for Mental Hygiene," which states, "The Nova Scotia Hospital has been in desperate need of staff for many years now . . . The hospital exists as a training center for the professions of psychiatry, social work and psychology but seems unable to retain a sufficient proportion of these people to make the improvements in patient care that are necessary. The establishment of a rehabilitation and follow-up program is very necessary for the patient to make an adequate adjustment to the community and for him to continue in a state of good mental health. The staff at the hospital at the present time is not sufficient to carry out such a program and every effort should be made to rectify this situation.

13. "Report of the Scientific Planning Committee of the Nova Scotia Society for Mental Hygiene."

14. C. Marshall, "Nova Scotia's Mental Health Program, an Address in Reply to the Report . . . of the Scientific Planning Committee of the Nova Scotia Society for Mental Hygiene," mimeographed typescript, October 1955, p. 11.

15. The full text of the memo is given in Appendix B, with all proper names changed to code names. The words of the memo turned out to be prophetic. The Mental Health Administration never accepted them; and the Board never understood them. These two facts played a major part in the staff becoming filled with people for whom such ideas had little meaning. The Stirling County Study tried to maintain the benefits of research as an important consideration in the Centre's policy formation. This was not successful because once the Study relinquished its formal control of the Centre, its influence in policy matters began to fade. That fading was undoubtedly hastened by the fact that the Study, in order to encourage autonomy and self-reliance on the part of the Board, adopted a policy of noninterference and of retreat into the background.

16. For a discussion of research and service as complementary rather than as alternatives, see N. Sartorius, "Priorities for research likely to contribute to better provision of mental health care," *Social Psychiatry*, vol. 12, 1977, pp. 171–84.

17. The steps taken to choose the Advisory Board were influenced by previous experi-

ences of the Stirling County Study. Starting in 1948, the Study had assembled a panel of advisors by means of a systematic inquiry that identified influential and well-thought-of persons in the main population clusters of the county. These individuals were for the most part natives of the area in which they lived and had life histories which were deeply imbedded in its social structure. They had proved of immense value in guiding the sociological and anthropological field work and had greatly helped the field workers to secure the information and opportunities for observation they sought. It was our hope that the Centre's Board might be composed of similar people. Our knowledge of the leadership and influence patterns in Stirling County was utilized, therefore, in selecting some of the persons to whom the letter was sent. With regard to Harwich and Kingston Counties, however, we lacked comparable information.

8. The Bristol Centre: community participation

1. A. H. Leighton and A. Longaker, "The Psychiatric Clinic as a community innovation," in A. H. Leighton, J. A. Clausen, and R. N. Wilson, eds., *Explorations in Social Psychiatry*, New York, Basic Books, 1957, pp. 365–85.

2. One research aim of the Stirling County Study was to explore the hypothesis that disintegration led to increased rates of mental illnesses. This required an examination of integration and disintegration across the entire county with intensive investigation of certain selected focus areas. See C. Hughes, M. A. Tremblay, R. N. Rapport, and A. H. Leighton, *People of Cove and Woodlot*, New York, Basic Books, 1960.

3. A. J. Vidich and J. Bensman, "Small Town in Mass Society," reprinted in part in R. L. Warren, ed., *Perspectives on the American Community: A Book of Readings*, Chicago, Rand McNally, 1966, p. 208.

4. A. de Toqueville, "Democracy in America," reprinted in part in Warren, *Perspectives on the American Community*, p. 447.

5. C. I. Schottland, "Federal Planning and Local Planning Agencies," in Warren, *Perspectives on the American Community*, p. 293.

6. Vidich and Bensman, "Small Town in Mass Society," p. 210.

7. Warren, *Perspectives on the American Community*, p. 195.

8. C. Sower, J. Holland, K. Tiedke, and W. Freeman, "The Death of the Health Council," in Warren, *Perspectives on the American Community*, pp. 280–91.

9. Warren, *Perspectives on the American Community*, p. 199.

10. L. C. Kolb, "Against the Radical Position in Community Mental Health," in Harry Gottesfeld, ed., *The Critical Issues of Community Mental Health*, New York: Behavioral Publications, 1972, p. 55.

11. Warren, *Perspectives on the American Community*, p. 222.

12. A. H. Leighton, *My Name Is Legion: Foundations for a Theory of Man in Relation to Culture, Volume 1: The Stirling County Study of Psychiatric Disorder and Sociocultural Environment*, New York, Basic Books, 1959, pp. 226–75.

13. C. R. Wright and H. H. Hyman, "Voluntary Association Memberships of American Adults," in Warren, *Perspectives on the American Community*, p. 454.

14. F. Hunter, "The Organized Community and the Individual," in Warren, *Perspectives on the American Community*, p. 516.

15. Vidich and Bensman, "Small Town in Mass Society," p. 211.

16. The spread of urban and suburban people, together with their sentiments, to rural areas and beyond has been well summarized by Peter Steinhart in his essay "Once More into the Woods" (*Audubon*, September 1980, p. 5). He says: "A rural revival has swept the nation in the last decade . . . It's not just ordinary sprawl, the city spreading at its edges like ink spilled onto a blotter. 'Migrants today are shunning large metropolitan areas in favor of

small ones,' says Rand Corporation researcher Peter A. Morrison. In some cases, they are following industry as it flees the cities, finding a job with an electronics firm in Colorado or a drug manufacturer in Tennessee. In other cases, they're going far beyond commute distances. Assemblyline workers in Flint are winterizing summer cottages in Northern Michigan, moving their wives and children up, and becoming weekend fathers . . . 'It is a major and unprecedented change,' says Calvin Beale, U.S. Department of Agriculture researcher who observed nearly ten years ago that the rural areas were no longer exporting people to cities but importing them from the cities. Says University of Pennsylvania geographer Dan Vining, 'There's virtually no rural county in the country that is not receiving net in-migration. For the first time, there's nothing in an urban area that cannot be had in a rural area.'

"It is also a sudden trend. In the 1960's, metropolitan areas were gaining over half a million people a year, and of the nation's twenty-five largest urban areas, only Pittsburgh was losing population. At the same time, rural areas were losing 300,000 people a year. By 1974, ten of the metropolitan areas were declining and the rural areas were gaining 380,000 people a year.

"An alarming aspect of the migration is the huge amount of countryside being turned into urban landscape. In the 1960's, rural land was disappearing under tract and pavement at a rate of about a million acres a year. In 1978, it was going under at a rate of three million acres a year.

"There is more at stake here than open space and wildlife habitat. We are about to lose the last vestiges of our rural tradition. As city people move out into the country, they displace the very openness and individuality they seek.

"In 1902, H. G. Wells predicted that 'the passion for nature' and 'that craving for a little private imperium' would result in exactly this transformation. Declared Wells, 'The city will diffuse itself until it has taken up considerable areas and many of the characteristics of what is now country. The country will take itself many of the qualities of the city. The old antithesis will cease, the boundary lines will altogether disappear.'

"So, our rural revival may be a last hurrah. Jimmy Carter, our first farmer President since Washington, may also be our last. The great sorrow here may not be the loss of land or the loss, even, of the rural outlook. The great sorrow may be the failure of it all to provide us with a better place in which to live. Our experience with the suburbs ought to suggest that flight from the cities only withdraws our commitment to solve urban problems and moves those problems out into the country."

17. Robert K. Merton, "Local and Cosmopolitan Influentials," in Warren, *Perspectives on the American Community,* pp. 254–8, 262.

18. The tabulations are based on two sources: the minutes of Board meetings and information gathered and observations made by Judge Cardoza and myself. Either Cardoza or I, or both of us, attended all but a very few Board meetings from the inception of the Advisory Board in 1956 until the end of March 1972. We already knew personally or grew acquainted with most of the Board members, and we kept notes on our observations. The fact that we were studying the functioning of the Centre was, of course, known to Board, staff, and provincial government. It was mentioned in the memo written by one of the Centre's psychiatrists on November 24, 1955 (see Appendix B), during the period when the Board was being developed, and was later stipulated in a memorandum of understanding between the Board and Cornell University, the latter acting on behalf of the Stirling County Study. It is also implicit in the Board's own *Memorandum of Association* (see Appendix A) in which the objectives included accumulating knowledge and analyzing "information obtained by the Centre as a basis for research into local problems" and providing "opportunity for observation, instruction, and research in mental health matters." These words were written into the memorandum in order to accommodate the work of the Stirling County Study. Further, the

Board and the staff always knew that the Stirling County Study (and, in part, the Centre itself) was supported by granting agencies who expected it to write reports on research concerned with improving mental health services and that these reports would be in the public domain.

19. With the aid of the Board minutes and our notes, supplemented by memory, Cardoza and I went over a list of all Board members and classified each individual as active or nonactive.

20. The reader will recall that the Board's function was to meet at least four times a year and to conduct the business of operating the Centre (see Appendix A).

21. To achieve this classification, Cardoza and I went over our list of active members and sorted them according to Merton's descriptive definitions of cosmopolitan and local influentials. It was interesting to discover that in almost every case the distinction appeared unequivocal.

22. H. Gottesfeld, *The Critical Issues of Community Mental Health,* New York, Behavioral Publications, 1972, p. 3.

23. Cottrell, for instance, says that when in the "average American local community" an attempt is made to mobilize and coordinate the resources for a focused attack on some problem, then one quickly sees "such a welter of institutional rivalries, jurisdictional disputes, doctrinal differences, and lack of communication that effective joint action seems well beyond practical possibility. And the problem of original concern begins to appear relatively simple compared with that of rendering the community capable of coordinated collective action." See Leonard S. Cottrell, Jr., "The Competent Community," in Berton H. Kaplan, Robert N. Wilson, and Alexander H. Leighton, eds., *Further Explorations in Social Psychiatry,* New York, Basic Books, 1976, p. 195.

24. Henry A. Foley, *Community Mental Health Legislation,* Lexington, Mass., Lexington Books, D. C. Heath, 1975, p. 92.

9. The Bristol Centre: the Board and the process of governance

1. The fact that the public in general do not appreciate research, teaching, and prevention in the way they do services has been identified by Lalonde as a serious problem for the funding of these activities. See Marc Lalonde, *A New Perspective on the Health of Canadians – A Working Document,* Ottawa, Government of Canada, April 1974, p. 30.

2. Aubrey Lewis, "William Mayer-Gross: An appreciation," *Psychological Medicine,* vol. 7, 1977, pp. 12–13, 15–16.

3. Bradley Buell, as quoted in Ralph Littlestone, "Planning Mental Health," in Saul Feldman, ed., *The Administration of Mental Health Services,* Springfield, Ill. Charles C Thomas, 1975, p. 19.

4. Seymour R. Kaplan, "Community Participation," in Feldman, *Administration of Mental Health Services,* p. 235.

5. These illustrations have been altered to protect identities.

6. S. Weir Mitchell, "Address before the fiftieth annual meeting of the American Medico-Psychological Association, held in Philadelphia, May 16th 1894," *Journal of Nervous and Mental Disease,* vol. 21, no. 7, July 1894, pp. 419–20.

7. Rudolf Klein and Janet Lewis, *The Politics of Consumer Representation: A Study of Community Health Councils,* London, Centre for Studies in Social Policy, 1976, p. 167.

8. H. Gottesfeld, *The Critical Issues of Community Mental Health,* New York, Behavioral Publications, 1972, p. 263.

9. G. Bateson, D. D. Jackson, J. Haley, and J. Weakland, "Toward a theory of schizophrenia," *Behavioral Science,* vol. 1, 1956, pp. 251–64.

10. Clyde Marshall, "The Nova Scotia Mental Health Plan," *Canada's Mental Health,* Supplement no. 28, May 1962, p. 6.

11. American Psychiatric Association, *Delivering Mental Health Services, Needs, Priorities and Strategies,* Washington, D.C., 1975, pp. 24, 34.

12. Ontario Royal Commission, Inquiry into Civil Rights, 1968, quoted by R. B. Blishen, *Doctors and Doctrines: The Ideology of Medical Care in Canada,* Toronto, University of Toronto Press, 1969, p. 88.

13. Warren R. Paap, "Consumer-based boards of health centers: Structural problems in achieving effective control," *American Journal of Public Health,* vol. 66, no. 6, June 1978, pp. 578–82. This report is based on a combination of the author's personal experience and a review of the literature. Although it deals with health rather than mental health centers, many of the phenomena reported and inferences drawn parallel those in our case study.

For a literature review specifically focused on community mental health, see J. K. Morrison, S. Holdridge-Crane, and Jane E. Smith, "Citizen participation in community mental health," *Community Mental Health Review,* vol. 3, no. 3, May–June 1978, pp. 1, 2–9. Here, too, many parallels to and variations on the themes we saw unfold at the Bristol Mental Health Centre are evident.

10. The behavior of social systems

1. See note 16, Chapter 8.

2. Robert B. Edgerton, "Anthropology, Psychiatry and Man's Nature," in Iago Galdston, ed., *The Interface between Psychiatry and Anthropology,* New York, Brunner/Mazel, 1971, p. 48.

3. Quoted in George Rosen, *Madness in Society: Chapters in the Historical Sociology of Mental Illness,* New York, Harper & Row, 1969, p. 186.

4. The discussions of care-giving agencies and small groups are based in part on my observations in Stirling County and on those reported in *The Governing of Men* (by Alexander H. Leighton, Princeton, N. J., Princeton University Press, 1945) and *Human Relations in a Changing World* (by Alexander H. Leighton, New York, E. P. Dutton, 1949). It also, however, draws on the work of the following authors: C. Argyris, *Intervention Theory and Method,* Reading, Mass., Addison-Wesley, 1970; R. F. Bales, *Interaction Process Analysis: A Method for the Study of Small Groups,* Reading, Mass., Addison-Wesley, 1950; W. B. Bennis and H. A. Shepard, "A theory of group development," *Human Relations,* vol. 9, 1956, p. 415; W. R. Bion, *Experiences in Groups,* New York, Basic Books, 1961; H. R. Bobbit, Jr., R. H. Breinholt, R. H. Doktor, and J. P. McNaul, *Organization Behavior, Understanding and Prediction,* Englewood Cliffs, N.J., Prentice-Hall, 1974; S. Feldman, ed., *The Administration of Mental Health Services,* Springfield, Ill., Charles C Thomas, 1975; A. P. Hare, E. F. Borgotta, and R. F. Bales, eds., *Small Groups: Studies in Social Interaction,* revised edition, New York, Alfred A. Knopf, 1965.

5. Alexander H. Leighton, *My Name is Legion: Foundation for a Theory of Man in Relation to Culture, Vol. 1: The Stirling County Study of Psychiatric Disorder and Sociocultural Environment,* New York, Basic Books, 1959, pp. 133–87.

6. Leighton, *My Name Is Legion,* vol. 1, pp. 133–87.

7. Eichna in discussing medical education says *"The focus and first priority of medical school education is the patient.* In practice, not so. Individual interests place their own desires and concepts first . . . The pressure groups include students, faculty and society. Students who are not fully qualified are admitted to medical school. Students who do not know what medicine is and what is best for patients, have by their protests altered the content, the teaching methods, the evaluation procedures and the standards of competence of medical school education. Faculty distorts the principle. Personal interests take over, and each member insists that a certain specialty receive favored treatment. Teaching hospitals twist the principle toward manual execution and the use of technologic procedures. They give less thought to patients and little to the learning of medicine. Society, also uninformed, gets into the act. Legislatures mandate admission numbers and even curriculum content . . . Lay and physician groups, each advocating a special interest, urge further special curricular changes. Governmental bodies of non-physicians issue dicta that in effect tell physicians what they can and cannot do for patients. All the above influences have their own specific aims as first priority, not the patient's well-being.''

Eichna's perspective and the conceptual basis of his analysis are different from mine, but I think he deals with the same phenomena. See Ludwig W. Eichna, ''Medical school education, 1975–1979,'' *New England Journal of Medicine,* vol. 303, no. 13, September 25, 1980, p. 728.

8. C. Marshall, ''More for the mind, a review and comparison,'' *Canadian Psychiatric Journal,* vol. 9, no. 1, 1964, pp. 13–14.

9. W. Kornhauser, ''Power and Participation in the Local Community,'' *Health Education Monographs,* No. 6, 1959. Reprinted in R. L. Warner, ed., *Perspectives on the American Community: A Book of Readings,* Chicago, Rand McNally, 1966. See quotations from this work in Chapter 5.

11. Approaches to action

1. The societal subsystems that have been emphasized and discussed in this book are, of course, a highly selected handful chosen because the case study indicated that they were major influences. As the reader probably realizes, other potential influences, such as socioeconomic class and culture, have been given little space. This does not mean that they were disregarded by us in our research or were without importance, but it does mean that they failed to emerge in the case study as having influence comparable to the subsystems that have been described. No doubt in many situations socioeconomic and cultural factors have telling effects on the provision and acceptance of services. The attention given to these topics by other writers is certainly warranted. At the same time, our experiences with the Bristol Mental Health Centre suggest that there are also a number of other influences deserving of attention because of the effects they are capable of exerting.

2. Quoted more fully in Chapter 8. R. L. Warren, *Perspectives on the American Community: A Book of Readings,* Chicago, Rand McNally, 1966, p. 222.

3. Quoted from the Royal Commission on Health by B. R. Blishen, *Doctors and Doctrines: The Ideology of Medical Care in Canada,* Toronto, Toronto University Press, 1969, p. 130.

4. By definition, disintegration of a social system means malfunction of its constituent parts, with particular reference to communication and coordination. Like other processes, that by which rewards are distributed and attained becomes fragmented and inconsistent as failures in communication and coordination occur. The psychological reactions to the stresses of disintegration add further confusion, impulsiveness, and unpredictability. See Alexander H. Leighton, ''The erosion of norms,'' *Australian and New Zealand Journal of Psychiatry,* vol. 8, 1974, p. 223.

5. The President's Commission on Mental Health, *Report to the President,* Vol. 1, Washington, D. C., U.S. Government Printing Office, 1978, p. 26.

6. Quoted in Lionel Trilling, *Matthew Arnold,* New York, Columbia University Press, 1949, p. 264.

7. A. Lief, ed., *The Commonsense Psychiatry of Dr. Adolf Meyer,* New York, McGraw-Hill, 1948.

8. The same is true of clinical psychology. See, for instance, S. B. Sarason, *The Psy-*

chological Sense of Community: Prospects for a Community Psychology, San Francisco, Jossey-Bass, 1974.

9. The Canadian Mental Health Association, *More for the Mind: A Study of Psychiatric Services in Canada,* Toronto, The Canadian Mental Health Association, 1963, p. 42.

10. This discussion of community mental health center policies is based partly on conversations through the years with Robert Felix and other participants. In addition, I have drawn on Henry A. Foley, *Community Mental Health Legislation: the Formative Process,* Lexington, Mass., Lexington Books and D. C. Heath, 1975.

11. Maurice R. Stein, *The Eclipse of Community: An Interpretation of American Studies,* New York, Harper & Row (Harper Torchbooks), 1960, p. 329.

Martindale and Hanson, publishing in 1969, provide an example of a study focused on a specific town that comes to similar conclusions: "In the twentieth-century world the Jeffersonian ideal of autonomous small towns has become anachronistic. Power is shifting from the locality to the great centers of government, industry and finance. If the small town survives at all it is not as an autonomous center of local life, but as a semidependent agency of distant power centers." D. Martindale and R. G. Hanson, *Smalltown and the Nation: The Conflict of Local and Translocal Forces,* Westport, Conn., Greenwood Publishing, 1969, p. xiv.

12. The President's Commission, *Report to the President,* pp. 5, 14–17, 43.

13. There are, of course, exceptions. Lee Robins and John Whiting are examples of a sociologist and an anthropologist whose work is quantitative and is known to many clinicians.

14. Foley, *Community Mental Health Legislation,* pp. 2–9, 65, 135–42. See also Joint Commission on Mental Illness and Health, *Action for Mental Health: Final Report of the Joint Commission on Mental Illness and Health,* New York, Basic Books, 1961, p. 284.

15. As is well known, Dorothea Dix based much of her argument for state and provincial hospitals on the bad treatment usually provided when the responsibility was local. The same point was made by Workman in writing about Upper Canada. He believed that the provincial hospitals served to protect the insane from the "niggardly economy" of "town and country" that strove to maintain them at the "lowest possible cost" resulting in harsh treatment and unclean living conditions. See Benjamin Workman, "Asylums for the chronic insane in upper Canada," *American Journal of Insanity,* vol. 24, July 1867, p. 47.

16. For a summary of some of the consequences, see S. A. Kirk and M. E. Therrien, "Community mental health myths and fate of former hospitalized patients," *Psychiatry,* vol. 38, August 1975, pp. 209–17.

17. This is evident in R. Robinson, D. F. DeMarche, and M. K. Wagle, *Community Resources in Mental Health,* New York, Basic Books, 1960.

18. Leonard S. Cottrell, Jr., "The Competent Community," in Burton H. Kaplan, Robert N. Wilson, and Alexander H. Leighton, eds., *Further Explorations in Social Psychiatry,* New York, Basic Books, 1976, pp. 195–209.

19. There are other parallel issues of equal importance that will not be discussed here because they were not prominent in the case study. Two, however, may be mentioned. The first is the potential conflict between excellence of patient care and a policy of maximizing professional opportunity for minority group members. This conflict, of course, is not inherent but comes when haste leads to appointing minority members who are not yet ready for the task. The second is the conflict between the desire for excellence in patient care and the desire to cut costs.

20. My aim is not simply to repeat for mental illness care in North America what John Lister and many others have said about Britain's national health services: "The years of expansion seem to be past, and the chill reality . . . that the demands upon the NHS are infinite whereas the resources are finite is at last being recognized." John Lister, "By the

London post," *New England Journal of Medicine,* vol. 302, no. 2, 1980, p. 102. Many people now appreciate that we are in a comparable situation. What I should like to emphasize consists of three points: (1) that the philosophy and goals of mental illness care have been out of line with resources since their inception almost two hundred years ago; (2) that the reason for this is that they were conceived and perpetuated in ignorance of the magnitude of the problem as reflected in actual prevalence rates; and (3) that the most immediate need is the same as has existed all along, namely, a rational set of priorities.

21. Joint Commission, *Action for Mental Health;* Canadian Mental Health Association, *More for the Mind;* M. Beiser, R. Krell, T. Lion, and M. H. Miller, eds., *Today's Priorities in Mental Health – Knowing and Doing,* Miami, Symposia Specialists, 1978; President's Commission, *Report to the President.*

22. American Psychiatric Association, *Diagnostic and Statistical Manual of Mental Disorders* (third edition), Washington, D.C., American Psychiatric Association, 1980.

23. Joint Commission, *Action for Mental Health,* p. 288.

24. Joint Commission, *Action for Mental Health,* p. 246.

25. Writing from the overview available to the World Health Organization's Division of Mental Health, Sartorius has provided an exceedingly lucid treatment of various factors involved in developing a frame of reference. He is concerned with the complementarity of research and service and with criteria for priorities, both those intrinsic to and those extrinsic to but affecting the mental illness field. It is interesting to see how many of his conclusions are translatable into the particulars observed in our case study of a single mental health service. N. Sartorius, "Priorities for research likely to contribute to better provision of mental health care," *Social Psychiatry,* vol. 12, 1977, pp. 171–84.

26. President's Commission, *Report to the President,* pp. 36–40.

27. Joint Commission, *Action for Mental Health,* see especially pp. 229–44 in reference to the discussion that follows.

28. Joint Commission, *Action for Mental Health,* p. 87.

29. Canadian Mental Health Association, *More for the Mind;* B. A. Martin, H. B. Kedward, and M. R. Eastwood, "Hospitalization for mental illness: Evaluation of admission trends from 1941 to 1971," *Canadian Medical Journal,* vol. 115, August 21, 1976, p. 325.

30. President's Commission, *Report to the President,* vol. 1, pp. 8, 17, 46, 49, vol. 2, pp. 144–220.

31. Although nonuse and abuse of science is very high in the mental illness field, it is far from being peculiar to this line of endeavor. Rather it is a particularly obtrusive example of a much more general hiatus between the requirements for applying science and the orientations of the public, the media, political representatives, and government agencies. This is well illustrated in the tragedy of the Love Canal at Niagara in New York. This was a dry trench that was first employed for dumping chemical wastes and then later covered over and used for building houses. As summed up by *The Lancet* (no. 8186, vol. 2, July 19, 1980, p. 132): "An early discovery by officials of the State Department of Health was a high rate of miscarriages among people living in the immediate vicinity. Elaborate questionnaires were used, directed to all those factors, environmental and personal, which might conduce to miscarriages. It was found that from 1958 to 1963 (and most houses were not built till the late '60's and early 70's) in those living nearest the dump site the miscarriage rate was 50%, as against an expected rate of 15%. This justified the earlier emergency action in which 200 families living near the dump site had been relocated. It was also found that by 1970 the local miscarriage rate had fallen to the expected, suggesting that whatever factor was responsible had disappeared. Television and the newspapers heightened the alarm of those still living in the vicinity of the Love Canal, and there was mounting pressure for either State or federal funds to evacuate and relocate hundreds of people. Alarm was increased when some local

scientists, from an inadequate study, concluded that local residents showed evidence of peripheral nerve damage. The claim was loudly proclaimed, but when it was withdrawn this passed almost unnoticed.

"Into this confused scene now came the lawyers from the Justice Department, who are preparing massive lawsuits against the Hooker [chemical] corporation. The State Health Department called for and planned an investigation of the chromosome patterns of local residents, only to find its proposals negated on the grounds of expense. The proposed study would have used adequate controls. The lawyers of the Justice Department then commissioned a chromosome study via the E.P.A. [Environmental Protection Agency]. This body put the matter in the hands of a private laboratory whose director had resigned over disputed results of a previous study of chromosome damage in which no controls had been used. Nor were they used in the Love Canal Study. Certain persons, 36 in all, were selected on the basis, it seems, that they would be likely to have abnormal chromosomes, having had children with birth defects or who developed cancer; and it was claimed that 11 of these had chromosomal defects conducive to malformations and cancer. The reaction was near-hysteria, and as a result the Federal Government has declared an emergency and agreed to relocate some 700 families, at least temporarily. In view of the alarm generated by the E.P.A. report there was indeed no alternative.

"It soon became evident that the report was worthless. Experts from the State Health Department and a panel set up by the Department of Health and Human Services criticized the report both because of the lack of controls and because of its scientific inadequacy. Finally, under great pressure, the E.P.A. set up a panel who examined the slides and could see no supernumerary acentric chromosome fragments. The members found no evidence that the Love Canal residents have excessive chromosome abnormalities, not even enough evidence to justify a larger study.

"It seems that the Justice Department lawyers who called for the chromosome survey were not prepared to put up either the time or the expenses of a full controlled study; they sought quick ammunition for their suit against the Hooker Corporation. In so doing they have profoundly depressed the standing of the E.P.A. If this were the last sin of the Justice Department it would be bad enough – but there is more to it. The survey made in 1978, which revealed the high miscarriage rate and also suggested a higher incidence of birth defects and low birth weights in 1958–62, was done as a careful scientific study and the respondents were promised that the confidentiality of records would not be violated; the survey involved over 3000 people, 'all their good habits and their bad ones, life styles, health, mental illnesses.' The Federal Government via the Department of Justice is now demanding that all this information be turned over to assist its suits against the Hooker Corporation."

32. Marc Lalonde, *A New Perspective on the Health of Canadians: A Working Document,* Ottawa, National Health and Welfare, Government of Canada, 1974, p. 57.

33. Consider the following protest against the development of a generally accepted psychiatric nosology: "The point is that totalitarianism does *not* yet exist in psychiatry. There are different models and concepts of what constitutes schizophrenia, or manic-depressive illness, and many other things, and who is to say that it is Dr. Wing, or Dr. Winokur, or Dr. Liang, or Dr. Schneider or anyone else who has, or had, the 'right answer.' " J. Berger, "Review of *Psychiatry in Dissent: Controversial Issues in Thought and Practice,*" *Canadian Journal of Psychiatry,* vol. 24, no. 1, February, 1979, p. 96. Berger's point of view ignores not only the history of science and the purpose of its scientific terms but also a much earlier biblical lesson. When the Lord wished to stop the building of a tower toward heaven, he made everyone speak a different language.

34. A. B. Hollingshead and F. C. Redlich, *Social Class and Mental Illness: A Community Study,* New York, John Wiley, 1958.

35. Marc Lalonde, *A New Perspective on the Health of Canadians,* 1974, p. 69.

36. *The Lancet,* no. 8150, vol. 2, November 10, 1979, p. 1000.

Index

Acadia Institute, 123
Acadia University, 56, 69, 123
Action for Mental Health (Joint Commission on Mental Illness and Health, U.S.), 70–1, 217, 226
Adamson, Elizabeth I., 48
Adler, Alfred, 40, 210
affect, concept of, 10
agencies, care-giving, 179–82, 199–200
  charitable service policies in, 182
  covert resistance in, 182
  division of responsibilities in, 217–19
  goals disregarded in, 179, 200
  governance of, 181–2, 214–16, 218, 220, 230
  as hostage to staff, 181, 189–90
  impact of social disintegration on, 182, 200, 215, 263n4
  interagency cooperation among, 217–18
  in local social crises, 219–20
  manipulative management in, 182
  motivations of individuals in, 186–7, 215
  nonalignment of goals and resources in, 180, 200, 216, 264n20
  priorities in, 216–17, 220
  private service policies in, 182
  recognition and rewards in, 186–7, 200, 215–16, 218
  resource inadequacy in, 200, 216
  staff problems in, 180–1, 200
  as subsystems of society, 179, 183, 199–200
  survival as first imperative of, 179–80, 181, 200
  troika characteristics of 181–2
  universal-service policies in, 180, 182
Alexander, Franz, 40
American Psychiatric Association, 47, 80, 171, 211
anomie, concept of, 44–5, 51
anthropology, 4, 37, 40, 42–4, 51, 120, 210

antipsychiatry, 80–1, 207
Aristotle, 178
Association for the Study and Prevention of Tuberculosis, 31
Atlee, Benge, 36–7
Aydelotte, Wm. O., x

Balkan Wars among disciplines, 11, 72–3
barriers, *see* mental health care barriers to
Baudelaire, C. P., 40
Beard, George Miller, 28
Beers, Clifford, 32, 33–4, 36, 250n51
Bell, Hugh, 24, 36 246n24
Belliveau, Robert, x
Benedict, Ruth, 40, 210
Bensman, J., 136, 137, 140
Bernheim, H., 30
Billings, Josh, 203
biological determinism
  cultural determinism vs., 43
  mental hospital movement vs., 13, 15, 20, 21, 27
  Meyer's rejection of, 30
  neurology and, 28
Bismark, von O. E., 18
Black, Douglas, x
Black, John, x
Blackmer, A. R., 82, 116–17
Bleuler, Eugen, 38
Blishen, R. B., 75–6, 115, 116
Borus, Jonathan F., 74
Bowlby, John, 42
Bremer, J., 13, 226
Brennan, Donald, x
Brison, Eliza, 36
Bristol Mental Health Centre
  academic collaboration as goal of, 63; 68–9, 113, 114, 159–160
  Bylaws, 234
  case studies (clinical) as a goal of, 61, 67
  case study of the Centre, 1–4, 83, 196